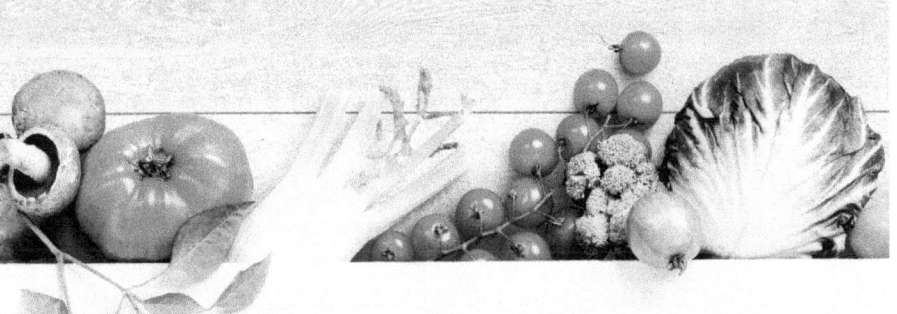

Fatty Liver and Cirrhosis Diet Cookbook

300 days of delicious recipes to manage hepatic conditions

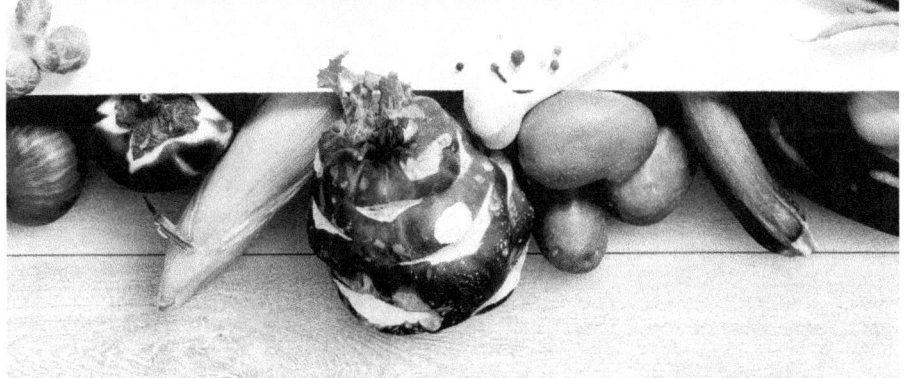

Appreciation

Hey there!
Just a quick note before you progress to the delicious recipes: I want to express my sincere appreciation for picking up this book. Taking charge of your health, especially your liver health, is a powerful decision, and I'm here to support you every step of the way. This book is packed with information and recipes to help you navigate a liver-friendly lifestyle, but remember, you're not alone on this journey. If you have questions, you can send me an email, or if you simply want to share your progress, don't hesitate to reach out!

chatwithlayla77@gmail.com

Copyright © 2024 by Layla Gael

All rights reserved. No part of this book may be reproduced, stored, or transmitted by any means whether auditory, graphic, mechanical, or electronic without written permission of both the publisher and the copyright owner of this book, except in the case of brief quotations embodied in critical articles and reviews. Unauthorized reproduction of any part of this work is illegal and is punishable by law.

The bonuses are located on page 84 and page 85 for the purchasers of this book

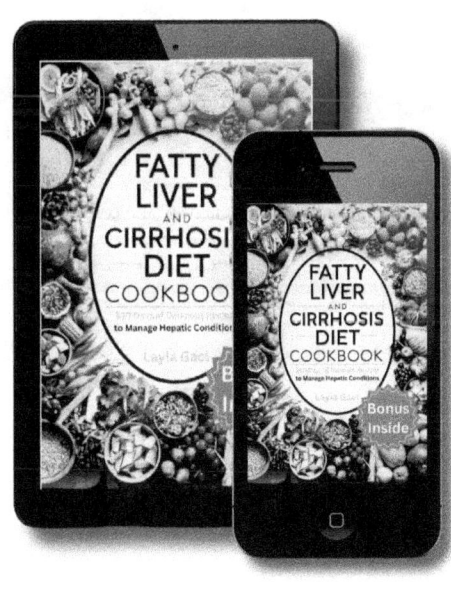

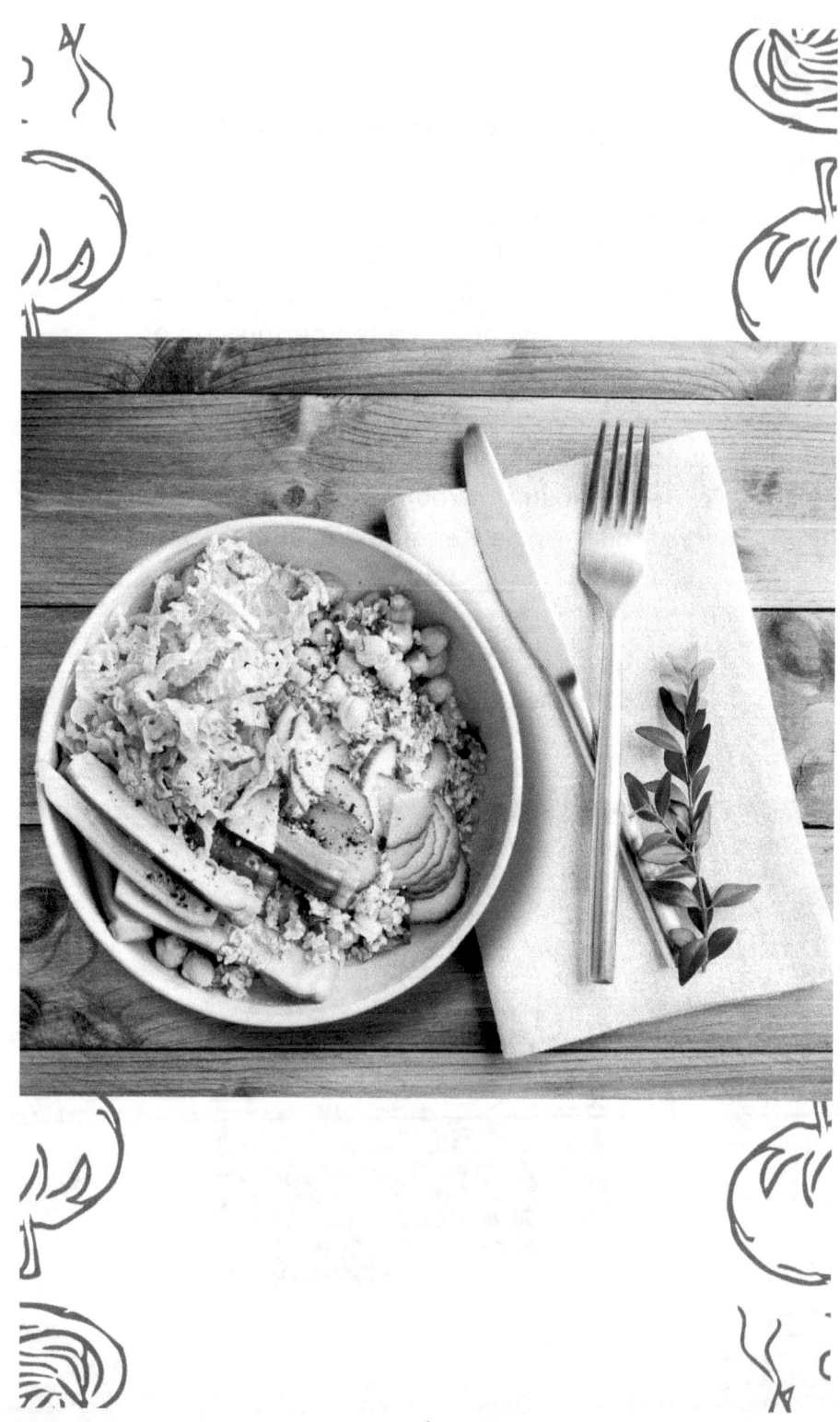

Table Of Contents

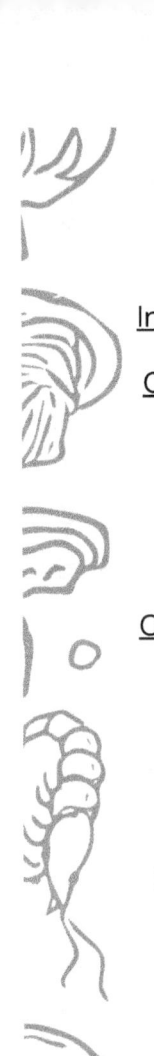

Introduction 9

Chapter 1: The Basics of Fatty Liver and Cirrhosis 13
    What is Fatty Liver Disease? 13
    Understanding Cirrhosis: Causes and Symptoms 13
    What prescription drugs can cause liver disease 15

Chapter 2: Scientific Insights and Research 17
    Latest Research on Fatty Liver and Cirrhosis 17
    Role of Nutrition in Preventing and Managing Liver Conditions 17
    Debunking Myths About Liver Health 20

Chapter 3: Types of Fatty Liver Conditions and Diets 23
    Non-Alcoholic Fatty Liver Disease (NAFLD): 23
    Alcoholic Fatty Liver Disease: 24
    Nutritional recommendations to mitigate the damage caused by alcohol consumption 25

Chapter 4: Understanding Your Liver: 27
    The Four Stages of Cirrhosis 27

Chapter 5: Managing Symptoms and Complications 29
    Symptom-Specific Management: 29

Chapter 6: Recipes 31
    Breakfast 31
    Whole-Wheat Toast with Smoked Salmon and Cream Cheese 31
    Berry Chia Seed Pudding 32
    Spicy Veggie Frittata 33

	High-Fiber Oatmeal with Apples and Cinnamon	34
	Scrambled Eggs with Avocado and Tomatoes	35
Lunch		36
	Tuna Salad with Whole-Wheat Pita and Vegetables	36
	Lentil Soup with Whole-Wheat Toast	37
	Greek Chicken Salad with Whole-Wheat Wrap	38
	Quinoa Salad with Roasted Vegetables	39
	Edamame Bowl with Brown Rice and Vegetables	40
Dinner		41
	Baked Salmon with Roasted Asparagus and Quinoa	41
	Chicken Stir-Fry with Brown Rice and Vegetables	42
	Turkey Meatloaf with Mashed Cauliflower	43
	Vegetarian Chili with Quinoa and Black Beans	44
	Lentil and Vegetable Soup with Whole-Wheat Bread	45
Snack		46
	Apple Slices with Almond Butter	46
	Cottage Cheese with Berries and Chia Seeds	47
	Edamame Pods with Sea Salt	48
	Roasted Chickpeas with Spices	49
	Greek Yogurt with Sliced Banana and Walnuts	50

Salads — 51

- Quinoa Salad with Roasted Vegetables and Feta — 51
- Arugula Salad with Pears, Walnuts, and Blue Cheese — 52
- Lentil Salad with Cucumber, Tomato, and Lemon Dill Dressing — 53
- Greek Salad with Grilled Chicken and Lemon Oregano Vinaigrette — 54
- Tuna Salad with Celery, Grapes, and Walnuts — 55

Soups — 56

- Lentil Soup with Lemon and Herbs — 56
- Tomato and Basil Soup with Whole Wheat Croutons — 57
- Chicken Noodle Soup with Vegetables — 58
- Curried Butternut Squash Soup with Coconut Milk — 59
- Split Pea Soup with Lemon and Mint — 60

Stews — 61

- Mediterranean Chickpea Stew with Tomatoes and Spinach — 61
- Turkey and Vegetable Stew with Brown Rice — 62
- Beef and Butternut Squash Stew with Whole Wheat Couscous — 63
- Lentil and Mushroom Stew with Barley — 64
- Chicken and White Bean Stew with Kale — 65

Fish Recipes — 66

- Baked Cod with Lemon and Herbs — 66
- Tuna Salad with Whole Wheat Crackers and Vegetables — 67
- Pan-Seared Salmon with Garlic and Spinach — 68
- Poached Tilapia with Vegetables and Dill Sauce — 69
- Baked Haddock with Tomato and Herbs — 70

Dessert 71
    Baked Apples with Cinnamon and Walnuts 71
    Frozen Banana "Nice Cream" 72
    Baked Pears with Ginger and Spices 73
    Greek Yogurt Parfait with Berries and Granola ... 74
    Dates with Nut Butter and Dark Chocolate 75

Vegetable 76
    Roasted Brussels Sprouts with Balsamic Glaze ... 76
    Sautéed Green Beans with Garlic and Almonds ... 77
    Steamed Asparagus with Lemon and Herbs 78
    Roasted Butternut Squash with Cinnamon and Pecans ... 79
    Sauteed Zucchini with Tomatoes and Basil 80

Chapter 7: 7-Day Sample Meal Plan 81
Bonus: Free Audio Version 84
Bonus: 21-Day Meal Planner 85-105
Chapter 8: Lifestyle Changes for Liver Health 107
    Importance of Regular Exercise in Managing Liver Conditions ... 107
    Stress Management Techniques for Liver Wellness ... 108
    Tips for Limiting Alcohol Consumption 109
    Foods and fruits to take and to avoid 110
    Natural Methods to Detoxify the Liver 115

Conversion chart 118
Conclusion 119

Introduction

The 12th most common cause of death in the US is liver cirrhosis.
1.48 million deaths were caused by cirrhosis in 2019.
Fatty liver disease has become a growing concern worldwide. According to recent data, the prevalence of fatty liver disease has been on the rise, affecting millions of individuals globally.

This increase is closely linked to the surge in obesity rates and unhealthy lifestyles, including sedentary behavior and poor dietary habits. Alarmingly, fatty liver disease can progress to more severe conditions such as liver cirrhosis and liver cancer if left untreated. As such, there is an urgent need for public health interventions and increased awareness to address this silent epidemic.

In our family's past, there's a story that changed how we see health. It started with a rumor about a relative who got very sick with a liver problem called fatty liver disease. Even though we didn't know all the details, we knew it was serious—it led to end-stage liver cirrhosis, a really bad stage of the lillness, which eventually ended up with him getting a liver transplant.

This scared us a lot. So when we heard that my distant cousin also had fatty liver disease, we didn't waste any time. We jumped into action, determined to help him.

Since my parents weren't around, I took care of my uncle. I made sure he ate right and went to all his doctor appointments on time.

But it wasn't just about fixing his body; it was also about giving him hope and strength. With help from doctors and our family, my uncle started to get better. It wasn't easy, but we never gave up.

Regular check-ups became a part of our routine, reminding us how important it is to take care of ourselves. And over time, my uncle got stronger and healthier.

Now, when I think back on everything we went through, I remember how vital it is to pay attention to our health and take action when something's wrong. Our journey with fatty liver disease was tough, but it showed us the power of hope, strength, and love.

Alright, listen up. Fatty liver and cirrhosis ain't no joke. We're talking about serious conditions that can wreak havoc on your health if you don't take them seriously. Fatty liver? It's like your liver's drowning in fat, and if you don't do something about it, it could lead to some major issues down the road. And cirrhosis? That's when your liver gets scarred up real bad, and trust me, you don't want that. It can mess with your whole body and even be life-threatening. So, yeah, paying attention to your liver health? It's kind of a big deal.

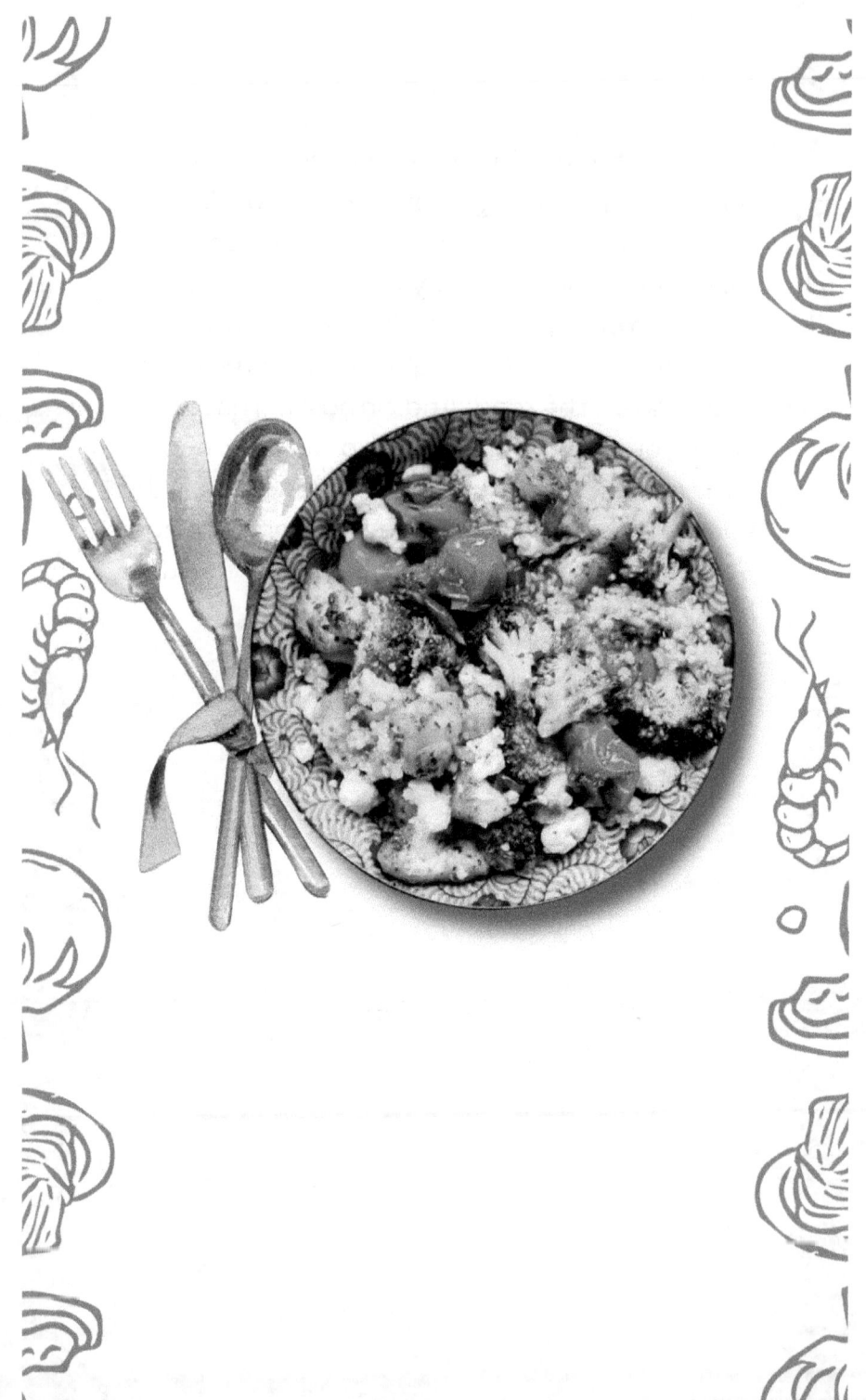

Chapter 1: The Basics of Fatty Liver and Cirrhosis

What is Fatty Liver Disease?

Fatty liver is when your liver starts hoarding fat like it's going out of style. Now, a little fat in there is normal, but when it piles up too much, that's when trouble starts brewing. It's often linked to things like obesity, diabetes, and high cholesterol. But here's the kicker: you might not even know you have it because it doesn't always cause symptoms. Sneaky, right? But don't let that fool you.

Fatty liver can lead to some serious issues like liver inflammation and scarring, which can eventually progress to cirrhosis if you're not careful. So, if you're feeling sluggish or have unexplained weight gain, it might be worth getting checked out. And remember, a healthy lifestyle with a balanced diet and regular exercise can go a long way in keeping your liver happy and fat-free.

Understanding Cirrhosis: Causes and symptoms

Let's dig deeper into understanding cirrhosis. Cirrhosis is like the grand finale of liver damage, where your liver becomes scarred and hardened due to long-term injury. Liver cirrhosis can come from various sources, such as excessive alcohol intake, chronic infections like hepatitis, fatty liver or certain medications. Over time, these attacks take their toll, leaving your liver riddled with scars.

Now, let's talk about symptoms. Cirrhosis doesn't exactly announce its arrival with fireworks. Instead, it's more like a silent intruder, creeping into your life with subtle signs. You might notice persistent fatigue, loss of appetite, or jaundice, where your skin and eyes take on a yellowish hue.

Catching cirrhosis early can make all the difference. So if you're experiencing any of these symptoms, don't brush them off. Get yourself checked out pronto. And remember, prevention is key. Cutting back on alcohol, maintaining a healthy diet, and staying on top of any underlying health conditions can help keep your liver in tip-top shape.

What prescription drugs can cause liver disease

Antibiotics: Certain antibiotics, like amoxicillin-clavulanate or erythromycin, can cause liver damage in some individuals.

Anti Seizure medications: Some medications used to control seizures, like phenytoin, can have side effects on the liver.

Antifungal medications: Some antifungal medications like ketoconazole can affect the liver negatively.

NSAIDs: Non steroidal anti-inflammatory drugs (NSAIDs) like ibuprofen, if used for long periods or at high doses, can potentially damage the liver.

Other prescriptions that can cause liver disease or liver damage include :

- Amiodarone.
- Anabolic steroids.
- Birth control pills.
- Chlorpromazine.

- Halothane (a type of anesthesia)
- Methyldopa.
- Isoniazid.
- Methotrexate
- Griseofulvin
- Tamoxifen
- Valproate
- Excess acetaminophen

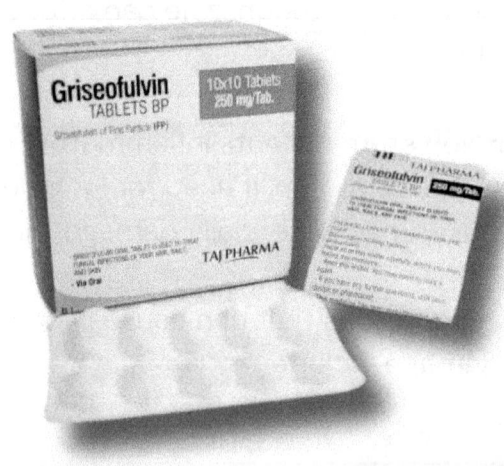

Chapter 2: Scientific Insights and Research

Latest Research on Fatty Liver and Cirrhosis

Recent research into fatty liver and cirrhosis unveils promising insights, blending modern science with ancient wisdom. Ayurveda, an ancient Indian system of medicine, offers holistic approaches to liver health. Studies reveal Ayurvedic herbs and therapies, such as milk thistle and turmeric, possess potent anti-inflammatory and hepatoprotective properties. These natural remedies complement conventional treatments, offering a multifaceted approach to managing liver conditions.

Role of Nutrition in Preventing and Managing Liver Conditions

In the quest for optimal liver health, nutrition emerges as a pivotal player, wielding the power to prevent and manage liver conditions with remarkable efficacy.

Increase Intake of Whole Grain Cereals

Whole grain cereals stand as stalwart guardians in the battle against liver conditions. Rich in fiber, vitamins, and minerals, they facilitate digestion and promote satiety, curbing the onslaught of unhealthy cravings and stabilizing blood sugar levels.

Don't Eat in Heavy Meals

Moderation emerges as the guiding principle when trying to maintain a healthy liver. Opting for smaller, more frequent meals alleviates the burden on the liver, allowing it to process nutrients with ease. Steer clear of heavy, indulgent feasts that tax the liver's resources and opt instead for light, balanced meals that nurture rather than overwhelm.

Stay Away from Fast Foods

Fast foods, laden with trans fats, refined sugars, and artificial additives, pose a grave threat to liver health. Their insidious allure may tempt the palate, but their detrimental effects on the liver are undeniable. resist the siren call of fast food establishments, opting instead for wholesome, home-cooked meals crafted with love and care.

Limit Intake of Meat

While meat may offer a rich source of protein, excessive consumption can burden the liver and predispose it to inflammation and damage. Exercise prudence and moderate your intake of red and processed meats, opting instead for leaner alternatives such as skinless poultry, fish, and plant-based proteins.

Avoid Salty Foods

Sodium-laden foods pose a double threat to liver health, elevating blood pressure and increasing the risk of fluid retention and liver damage. scrutinize food labels, choosing low-sodium alternatives and seasoning your meals with herbs and spices for flavor enhancement.

Debunking Myths About Liver Health

Myth 1: Fatty liver only affects heavy drinkers.

Fact: While alcohol abuse is a common cause, non-alcoholic fatty liver disease (NAFLD) affects those with poor diet and sedentary lifestyles.

Myth 2: Fatty liver is harmless and doesn't progress to cirrhosis.

Fact: Untreated fatty liver can progress to cirrhosis, a serious condition with irreversible liver damage.

Myth 3: Cirrhosis only affects older adults.

Fact: Cirrhosis can develop at any age, particularly in individuals with chronic liver conditions like hepatitis.

Myth 4: Liver cirrhosis is always caused by alcohol abuse.

Fact: Cirrhosis can also result from hepatitis, fatty liver disease, and other factors like genetic disorders or autoimmune diseases.

Myth 5: Liver cirrhosis is untreatable and inevitably leads to death.

Fact: Early detection, lifestyle changes, and medical treatments can slow the progression of cirrhosis and improve quality of life.

Myth 6: Only overweight individuals develop fatty liver.

Fact: Fatty liver can affect individuals of all body types, including those who appear thin but have poor dietary habits.

Myth: Fatty liver will go away on its own over time.

Fact: Once developed, fatty liver disease tends to be a progressive condition without intervention.

The fat buildup does not resolve spontaneously and may worsen over time. To stop the progression, treatment and lifestyle modifications are crucial.

Myth: A fatty liver does not affect other organs.

Fact: The entire body may be affected when the liver gets inflamed and damaged due to excess fat.
The liver plays a key role in hormone production, nutrient processing and detoxification. So impaired liver function can have wide-ranging effects.

Myth: The liver fully regenerates overnight.

Fact: While regenerative, severe damage takes time to heal.

Causes of fatty liver

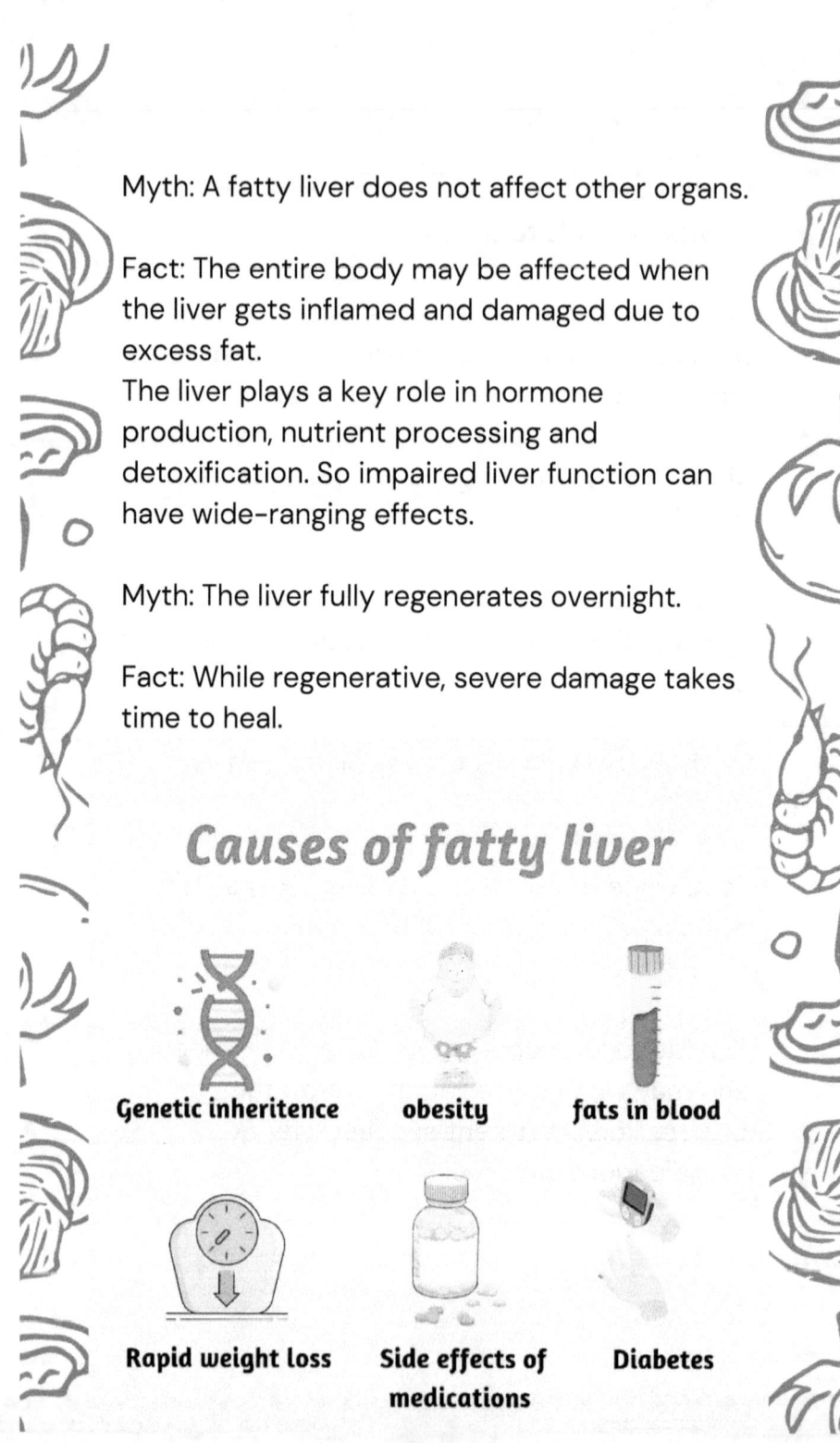

Genetic inheritence   obesity   fats in blood

Rapid weight loss   Side effects of medications   Diabetes

Chapter 3: Types of Fatty Liver Conditions and Diets

Non-Alcoholic Fatty Liver Disease (NAFLD):

Non-alcoholic fatty liver disease (NAFLD) is a prevalent liver condition characterized by excessive fat accumulation in the liver of individuals who consume little to no alcohol. It includes a range of disorders of the liver, from non-alcoholic steatohepatitis (NASH), which can lead to cirrhosis and liver failure, to simple fatty liver (steatosis).

Risk factors for NAFLD include obesity, insulin resistance, type 2 diabetes, and metabolic syndrome. Diagnosis typically involves blood tests, imaging studies, and sometimes liver biopsy to assess the severity of liver damage. Management strategies for NAFLD focus on lifestyle modifications, including weight loss, regular exercise, and dietary changes.

One effective dietary strategy to manage NAFLD is to implement a carbohydrate strategy known as carbohydrate cycling. This involves alternating between higher and lower carbohydrate intake days to optimize insulin sensitivity and fat metabolism. On higher carbohydrate days, focus on consuming complex carbohydrates from whole grains, fruits, and vegetables, while limiting simple sugars and refined carbohydrates. On lower carbohydrate days, emphasize lean protein sources, healthy fats, and non-starchy vegetables to promote fat burning and stabilize blood sugar levels. By incorporating carbohydrate cycling into your dietary regimen, you can effectively manage NAFLD and support liver health.

Alcoholic Fatty Liver Disease:

Alcoholic fatty liver disease (AFLD) is a condition characterized by the accumulation of fat in the liver due to excessive alcohol consumption. It is the earliest stage of alcohol-related liver disease and can progress to more severe conditions if not addressed. AFLD typically presents with no symptoms initially but can progress to inflammation (alcoholic hepatitis) and fibrosis (scarring of the liver), eventually leading to cirrhosis if alcohol consumption continues unabated. The liver's ability to function is impaired, impacting its vital roles in metabolism, detoxification, and nutrient storage.

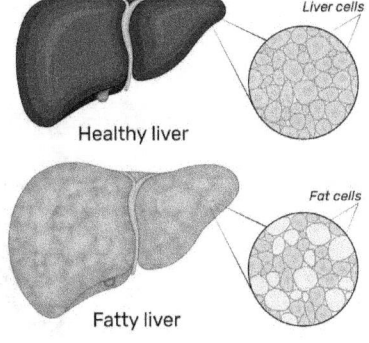

Nutritional recommendations to mitigate the damage caused by alcohol consumption

1. Increase intake of fruits and vegetables rich in antioxidants, such as berries, spinach, and broccoli, to combat oxidative stress.
2. Consume omega-3 fatty acids found in fatty fish like salmon and flaxseeds to reduce inflammation and support liver function.
3. Opt for lean sources of protein like poultry, legumes, and tofu to promote liver repair and regeneration.
4. Limit intake of processed foods, saturated fats, and added sugars, which can exacerbate liver damage.
5. Stay hydrated by drinking plenty of water to aid liver detoxification processes.

6. Avoid alcohol completely or limit intake to recommended levels to prevent further damage to the liver.

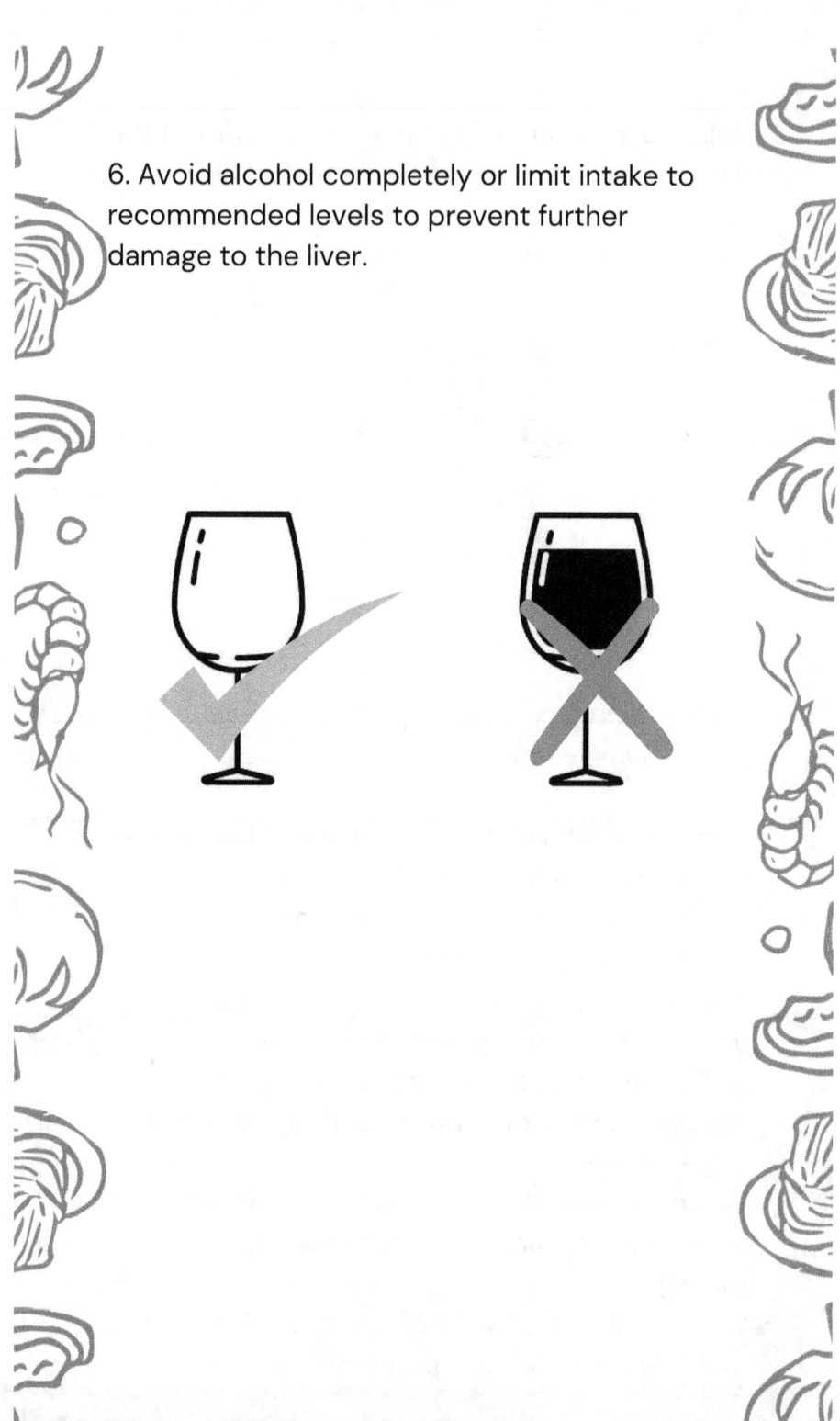

Chapter 4: Understanding Your Liver

The Four Stages of Cirrhosis

Steatosis (Fatty Liver): This is the initial stage where fat accumulates in the liver. It often has no symptoms and can be reversible with lifestyle changes.

Fibrosis : As inflammation persists, scar tissue (fibrosis) begins to develop in the liver. This stage might also have no symptoms, but it's a crucial point where intervention can prevent further progression.

Cirrhosis: When significant scarring replaces healthy tissue, liver function becomes impaired. This is cirrhosis, and as explained earlier, it's categorized based on compensated or decompensated function.

Liver Failure (End-Stage Liver Disease) : This is the most severe stage where the liver loses most of its function. It can lead to coma and death without a liver transplant.

Stages Of Cirrhosis

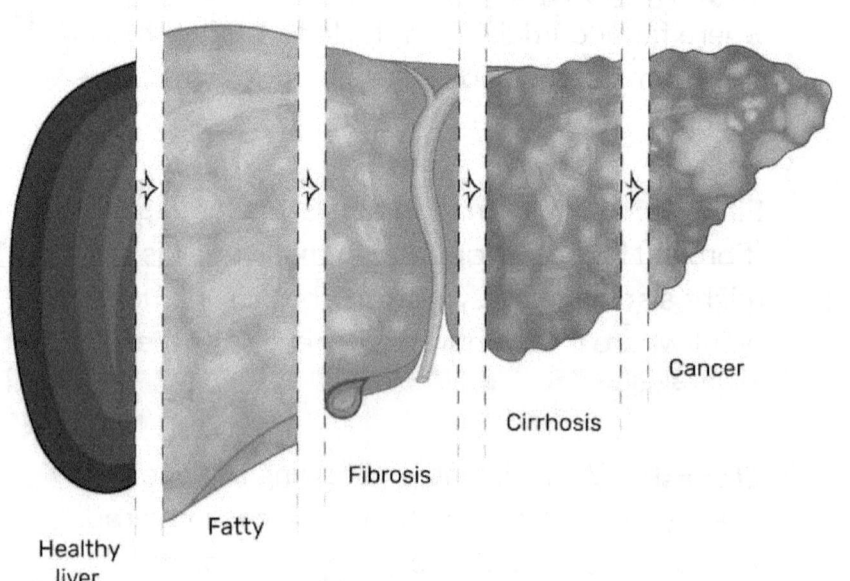

Healthy liver — Fatty — Fibrosis — Cirrhosis — Cancer

Chapter 5: Managing Symptoms and Complications

Symptom-Specific Management:

- Fatigue: Prioritize sleep, manage stress, and maintain a balanced diet with adequate protein intake. Doctors might recommend medications to manage fatigue in severe cases.

- Nausea and Vomiting: Smaller, frequent meals, avoiding greasy or spicy foods

- Itchy Skin: Moisturizers and medications can help alleviate itching.

- Ascites (abdominal swelling): Following a low-sodium diet and taking diuretics as prescribed are crucial. In severe cases, doctors might need to remove excess fluid with procedures like paracentesis.

- Confusion/ Hepatic encephalopathy: Hepatic encephalopathy is confusion and thinking problems caused by toxins building up from a failing liver. Lactulose, a medication, helps by drawing these toxins into the gut for removal.

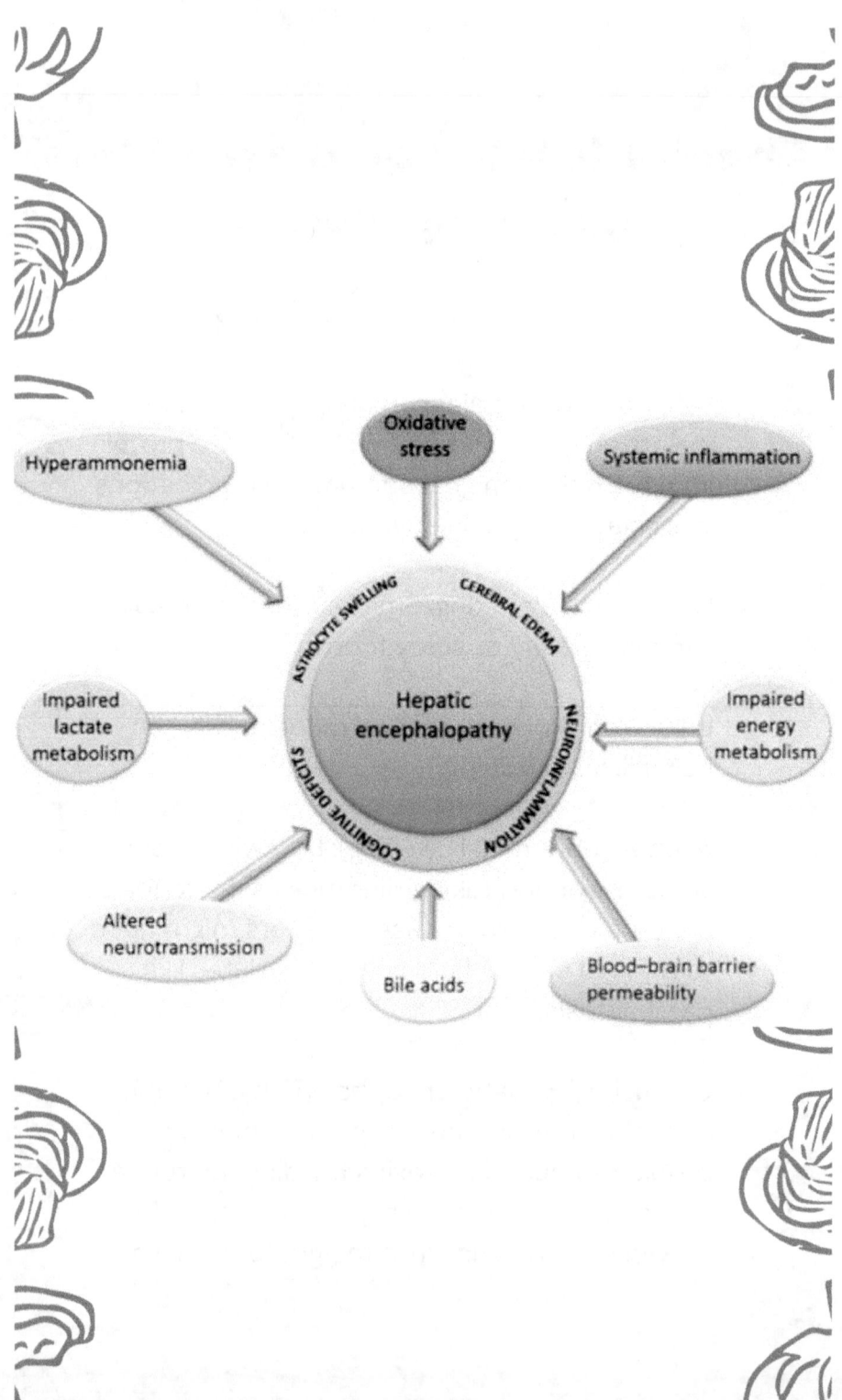

Chapter 6: Recipes

Breakfast

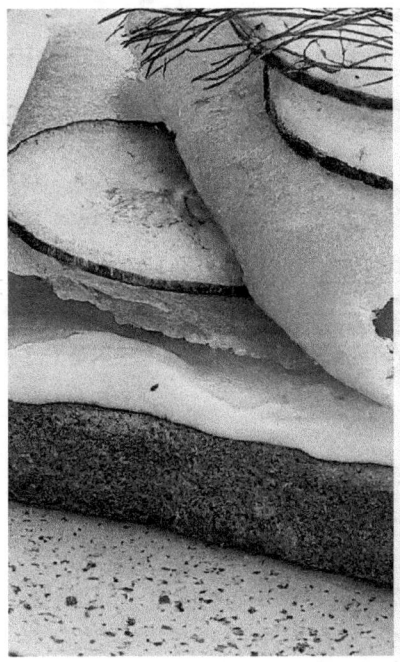

Whole-Wheat Toast with Smoked Salmon and Cream Cheese

 1 serving   10 minutes

INGREDIENTS
- 1 slice whole-wheat bread, toasted
- 2 ounces smoked salmon
- 1 tablespoon light cream cheese
- 1/4 cup sliced cucumber
- Fresh dill (optional)

DIRECTIONS

1. Toast the whole-wheat bread.
2. Spread the cream cheese on the toast.
3. Top with smoked salmon, cucumber slices, and fresh dill (optional).

NUTRITIONAL VALUE (APPROXIMATE):

- Calories: 250
- Protein: 18g
- Fat: 10g
- Carbs: 20g (fiber: 2g)

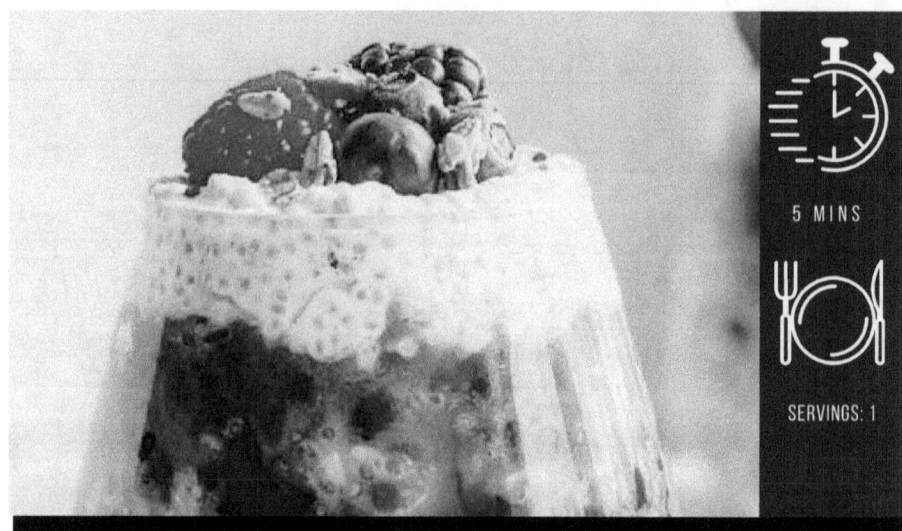

BERRY CHIA SEED PUDDING

5 MINS
SERVINGS: 1

INGREDIENTS

- 1/2 cup rolled oats
- 1/3 cup unsweetened almond milk
- 1/4 cup plain Greek yogurt (2% fat)
- 1/4 cup frozen mixed berries
- 1 tablespoon chia seeds
- 1/4 teaspoon vanilla extract (optional)

DIRECTIONS

1. In a jar or container, combine oats, almond milk, yogurt, berries, chia seeds, and vanilla extract (if using).
2. Stir well, cover, and refrigerate overnight.
3. In the morning, enjoy chilled.

NUTRITIONAL VALUE(APPROXIMATE):

- Calories: 300
- Protein: 12g
- Fat: 10g
- Carbs: 30g (fiber: 5g)

Spicy Veggie Frittata

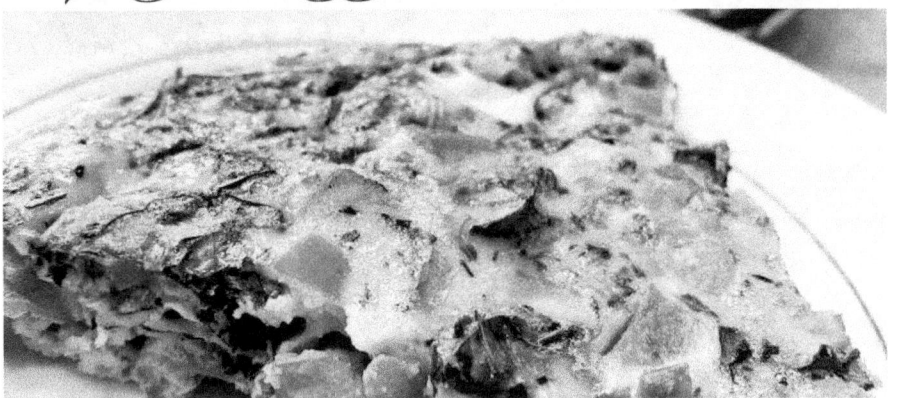

Ingredients:

- 4 eggs
- 1/2 cup chopped vegetables (bell pepper, onions, mushrooms)
- 1/4 cup chopped spinach
- 1/4 cup crumbled feta cheese
- 1 tablespoon olive oil
- Salt, pepper, and chili flakes (optional)

Instructions:

- Preheat oven to 375°F (190°C). Grease a small oven-safe pan.
- In a bowl, whisk together eggs with salt and pepper.
- In a pan, warm up the olive oil over medium heat.
- Add chopped vegetables and cook for 5 minutes, until softened.
- Stir in spinach and cook until wilted.
- Pour the egg mixture into the pan with vegetables.
- Sprinkle with feta cheese and chili flakes (optional).
- Bake in the preheated oven for 15-20 minutes, or until set.
- Serve warm or at room temperature.

Nutritional Value (Approximate):

Calories: 250
Protein: 12g
Fat: 15g
Carbs: 5g (fiber: 2g)

Servings: 2

Preparation time : 20 mins

High-Fiber Oatmeal with Apples and Cinnamon

★★★★☆

INGREDIENTS

1/2 cup rolled oats
1 cup unsweetened almond milk
1/2 apple, chopped
1 tablespoon ground flaxseed
1/4 teaspoon ground cinnamon
Pinch of salt (optional)

 1 serving 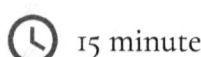 15 minutes

DIRECTIONS

1. In a saucepan, combine oats, almond milk, chopped apple, flaxseed, cinnamon, and a pinch of salt (optional).
2. Bring to a boil over medium heat.
3. Reduce heat and simmer for 5-7 minutes, or until oats are cooked through and desired consistency is reached.
4. Serve warm topped with additional chopped apple slices and a sprinkle of cinnamon (optional).

NUTRITIONAL VALUE (APPROXIMATE)

Calories: 300
Protein: 8g
Fat: 10g (healthy fats from flaxseed)
Carbs: 35g (fiber: 5g)

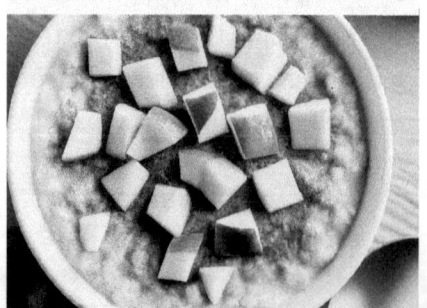

Scrambled eggs with avocado and tomatoes

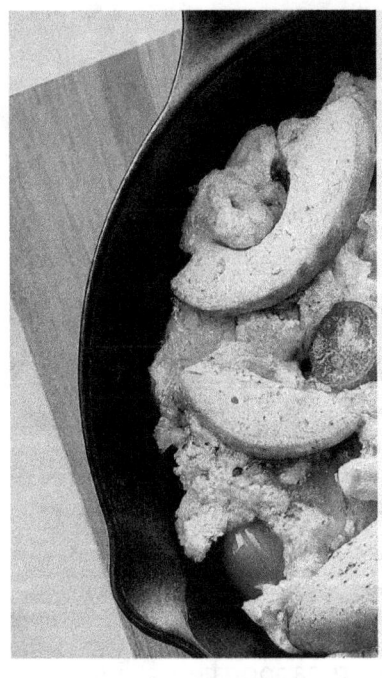

 1 serving   10 minutes

INGREDIENTS

2 large eggs
1/2 avocado, sliced
1/2 cup chopped tomatoes
1 tablespoon olive oil
Salt and pepper to taste
Optional: Finely chopped herbs that are fresh, such as chives or parsley

DIRECTIONS

- Beat eggs with a dash of pepper and salt in a bowl.
- In a pan, warm up the olive oil over medium heat.
- Add tomatoes and cook for 2-3 minutes, until softened slightly.
- Pour in the egg mixture and scramble until cooked through, to desired consistency.
- Serve immediately topped with sliced avocado and a sprinkle of fresh herbs (optional).

NUTRITIONAL VALUE (APPROXIMATE):
- Calories: 300
- Protein: 15g
- Fat: 18g (healthy fats from avocado and olive oil)
- Carbs: 5g (fiber: 2g)

Lunch

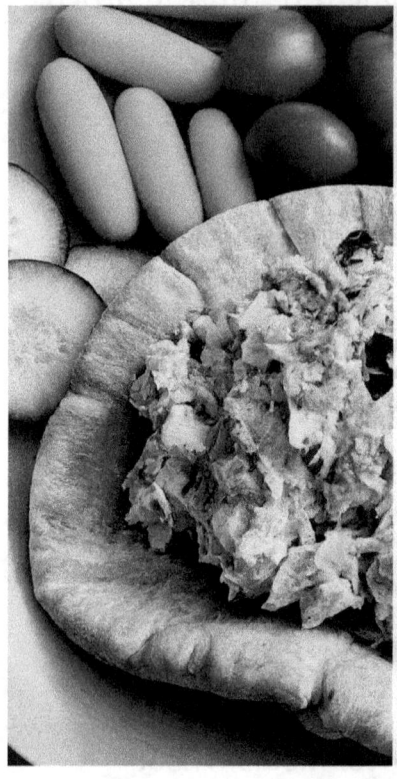

Tuna Salad with Whole-Wheat Pita and Vegetables

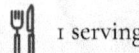 1 serving   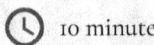 10 minutes

INGREDIENTS

1. 5 oz canned tuna in water, drained
2. 1 tablespoon light mayonnaise
3. 1 tablespoon chopped celery
4. 1 tablespoon chopped red onion
5. 1/4 teaspoon lemon juice
6. Salt and pepper to taste
7. 1 whole-wheat pita bread
8. Baby carrots, cherry tomatoes, and cucumber slices (for dipping)

DIRECTIONS

- In a bowl, combine tuna, mayonnaise, celery, red onion, lemon juice, salt, and pepper.
- Warm the whole-wheat pita bread according to package instructions (optional).
- Serve the tuna salad with the whole-wheat pita and vegetable sticks for dipping.

NUTRITIONAL VALUE (APPROXIMATE):

- Calories: 250
- Protein: 18g
- Fat: 10g
- Carbs: 20g (fiber: 2g)

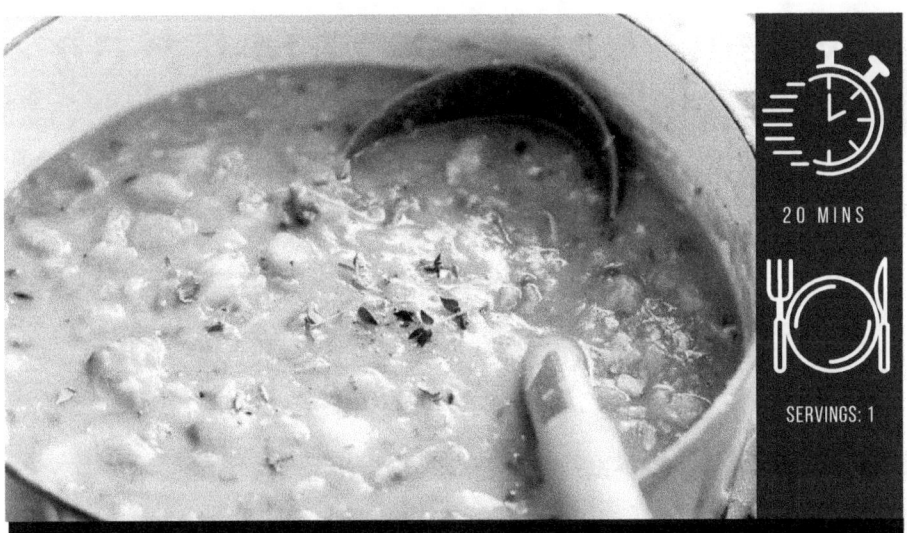

20 MINS

SERVINGS: 1

LENTIL SOUP WITH WHOLE-WHEAT TOAST

INGREDIENTS

- 1 cup cooked lentils (canned or pre-cooked)
- 2 cups vegetable broth
- 1/2 cup chopped vegetables (carrots, celery, onions)
- 1 clove garlic, minced
- 1 tablespoon olive oil
- 1/2 teaspoon dried thyme
- Salt and pepper to taste
- 1 slice whole-wheat bread, toasted

DIRECTIONS

1. Olive oil should be heated in a saucepan over medium heat.
2. Add chopped vegetables and cook for 5 minutes, until softened.
3. Cook for one more minute after adding the garlic.
4. Pour in vegetable broth, lentils, and thyme.
5. Bring to a boil, then reduce heat and simmer for 10-15 minutes, or until vegetables are tender.
6. Season with salt and pepper to taste.
7. Serve warm with a slice of whole-wheat toast.

NUTRITIONAL VALUE (APPROXIMATE):

- Calories: 300
- Protein: 15g
- Fat: 10g
- Carbs: 40g (fiber: 10g)

Greek Chicken Salad with Whole-Wheat Wrap

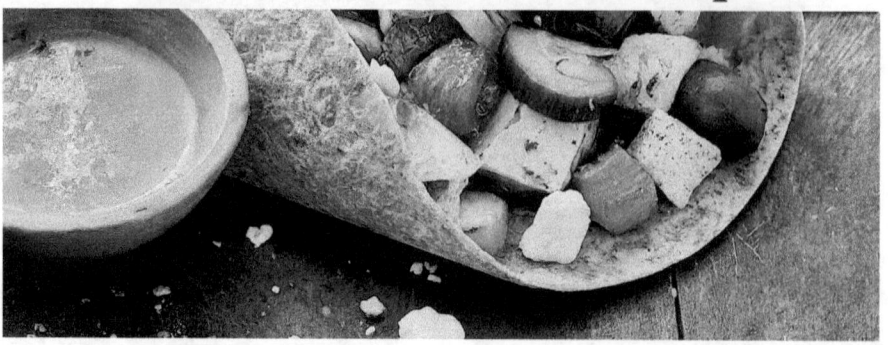

Ingredients:

- 3 oz grilled or baked chicken breast, chopped
- 1/4 cup crumbled feta cheese
- 1/4 cup chopped cucumber
- 2 tablespoons chopped tomatoes
- 1 tablespoon chopped red onion
- 1 tablespoon kalamata olives, chopped (optional)
- 1 tablespoon olive oil
- 1 tablespoon lemon juice
- 1/4 teaspoon dried oregano
- Salt and pepper to taste
- 1 whole-wheat wrap

Instructions:

- In a bowl, combine chopped chicken breast, feta cheese, cucumber, tomatoes, red onion, olives (optional), olive oil, lemon juice, oregano, salt, and pepper.
- Spread the salad mixture evenly in the center of a whole-wheat wrap.
- Roll up the wrap tightly.

Nutritional Value (Approximate):

Fat: 15g
Carbs: 5g (fiber: 2g)
Calories: 250
Protein: 12g

Servings: 1

Preparation time : 15 mins

Quinoa Salad with Roasted Vegetables

 1 serving   25 minutes

INGREDIENTS

1/2 cup cooked quinoa
1/2 cup roasted vegetables (broccoli, carrots, bell peppers)
1/4 cup chopped cucumber
1/4 cup cherry tomatoes
1 tablespoon crumbled feta cheese (optional)
1 tablespoon olive oil
1 tablespoon lemon juice
1/4 teaspoon dried basil
Salt and pepper to taste

DIRECTIONS

1. Preheat the oven to 400°F (200°C).
2. Toss chopped vegetables with a drizzle of olive oil and salt and pepper.
3. Roast vegetables in the preheated oven for 15-20 minutes, or until tender-crisp
4. While vegetables roast, cook quinoa according to package instructions.
5. In a bowl, combine cooked quinoa, roasted vegetables, chopped cucumber, cherry tomatoes, feta cheese (optional), olive oil, lemon juice, basil, salt, and pepper.
6. Serve chilled or at room temperature after tossing to coat.

NUTRITIONAL VALUE (APPROXIMATE)

- Calories: 350
- Protein: 10g
- Fat: 12g (healthy fats from olive oil)
- Carbs: 40g (fiber: 5g)

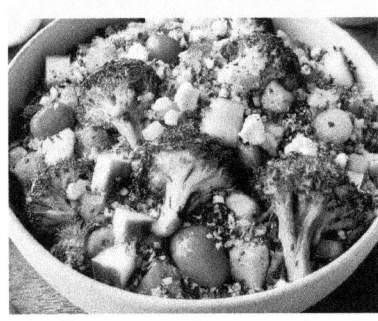

Edamame Bowl with Brown Rice and Vegetables

1 serving • 15 minutes

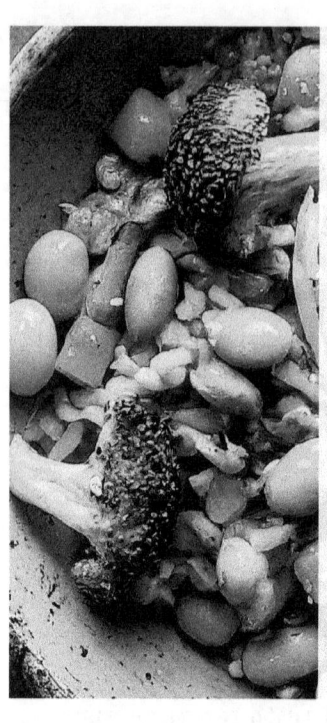

INGREDIENTS

1/2 cup cooked brown rice
1/2 cup shelled edamame, steamed or frozen
1/4 cup chopped carrots
1/4 cup chopped broccoli florets
1 tablespoon chopped red onion
1 tablespoon low-sodium soy sauce
1 teaspoon sesame oil
1/4 teaspoon grated ginger
Pinch of red pepper flakes (optional)
Sesame seeds for garnish (optional)

DIRECTIONS

1. Cook brown rice according to package instructions.
2. Steam or boil edamame according to package instructions, or thaw frozen edamame.
3. In a bowl, combine cooked brown rice, edamame, chopped carrots, broccoli, and red onion.
4. In a small bowl, whisk together soy sauce, sesame oil, ginger, and red pepper flakes (optional).
5. Shake to coat the salad after adding the dressing.
6. Garnish with sesame seeds (optional) and serve.

NUTRITIONAL VALUE (APPROXIMATE):

Calories: 350
Protein: 20g
Fat: 10g (healthy fats from sesame oil)
Carbs: 40g (fiber: 5g)

Dinner

Baked Salmon with Roasted Asparagus and Quinoa

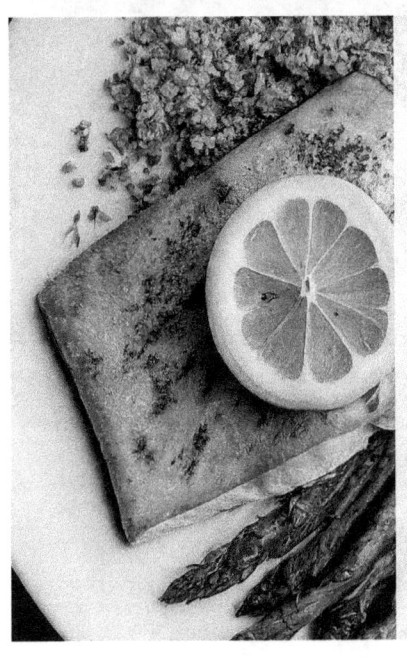

🍴 2 servings   🕐 45 minutes

INGREDIENTS

1. 2 salmon filets (4-6 oz each)
2. 1 bunch asparagus, trimmed
3. 1 cup cooked quinoa
4. 1 tablespoon olive oil
5. 1 tablespoon lemon juice
6. 1/2 teaspoon dried dill
7. Salt and pepper to taste

DIRECTIONS

- Preheat oven to 400°F (200°C).
- In a baking dish, toss asparagus with olive oil, salt, and pepper.
- Arrange salmon fillets on top of the asparagus.
- Whisk the dill and lemon juice together in a small bowl. Drizzle the mixture over the salmon.
- Bake for 20-25 minutes, or until salmon is cooked through and flakes easily with a fork.
- Serve with cooked quinoa.

NUTRITIONAL VALUE (APPROXIMATE):

- Calories: 400
- Protein: 30g
- Fat: 15g (healthy fats from salmon)
- Carbs: 35g (fiber: 5g)

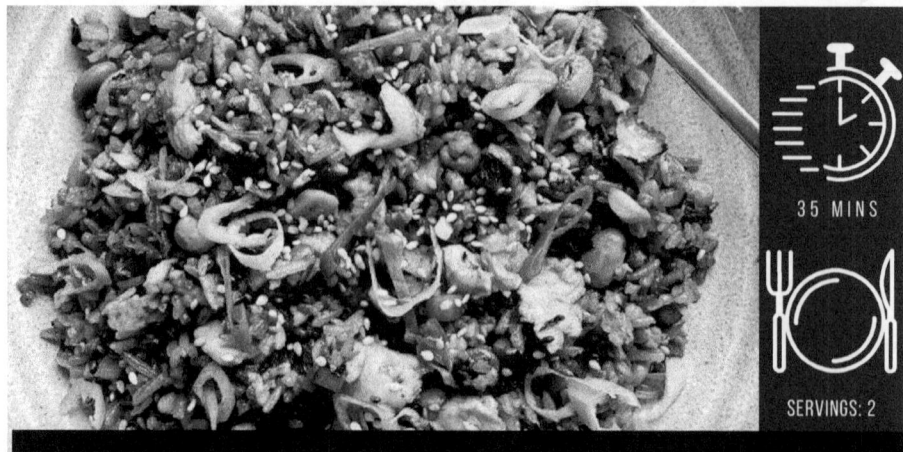

35 MINS

SERVINGS: 2

CHICKEN STIR-FRY WITH BROWN RICE AND VEGETABLES

INGREDIENTS

- 1 boneless, skinless chicken breast, sliced
- 1 cup chopped vegetables (broccoli, carrots, snap peas)
- 1/2 cup cooked brown rice
- 1 tablespoon low-sodium soy sauce
- 1 tablespoon rice vinegar
- 1 teaspoon cornstarch
- 1 tablespoon olive oil
- 1/2 teaspoon grated ginger
- Salt and pepper to taste

DIRECTIONS

1. In a small bowl, whisk together soy sauce, rice vinegar, cornstarch, and a splash of water to make a thin sauce.
2. In a big wok or skillet, warm up the olive oil over medium-high heat.
3. Cook the chicken for five to seven minutes, or until it turns brown.
4. Add chopped vegetables and cook for an additional 5 minutes, or until tender-crisp.
5. Pour the sauce mixture into the pan and cook for 1-2 minutes, or until thickened.
6. Serve stir-fry over cooked brown rice.

NUTRITIONAL VALUE(APPROXIMATE):

- Calories: 400
- Protein: 30g
- Fat: 10g
- Carbs: 40g (fiber: 5g)

Turkey Meatloaf with Mashed Cauliflower

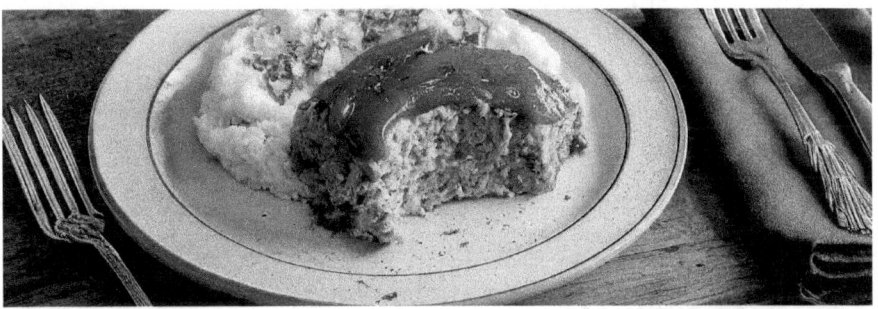

Ingredients:

1 pound lean ground turkey
1/2 cup chopped onion
1/4 cup chopped bell pepper
1/4 cup rolled oats
1 egg, beaten
1 tablespoon ketchup
1 tablespoon Worcestershire sauce
1/2 teaspoon dried thyme
Salt and pepper to taste
1 head cauliflower, cut into florets
Low-fat milk or unsweetened almond milk (for mashing)

Instructions:

- Preheat oven to 375°F (190°C).
- In a large bowl, combine ground turkey, onion, bell pepper, oats, egg, ketchup, Worcestershire sauce, thyme, salt, and pepper.
- After shaping the mixture into a loaf, transfer it to a baking dish.
- Bake for 25 minutes, or until cooked through.
- While the meatloaf bakes, steam or boil cauliflower florets until tender.
- Mash the cauliflower with a little low-fat milk or almond milk until desired consistency is reached.
- Serve meatloaf with mashed cauliflower.

Nutritional Value (Approximate):

- Calories: 400
- Protein: 40g
- Fat: 10g
- Carbs: 30g (fiber: 5g)

Servings: 4

Preparation time : 45 mins

INGREDIENTS

1 tablespoon olive oil
1 onion, chopped
2 cloves garlic, minced
1 bell pepper (any color), chopped
1 jalapeño pepper, seeded and chopped (optional)
1 (15 oz) can diced tomatoes, undrained
One fifteen-ounce can of rinsed and drained black beans
One fifteen-ounce can of washed and drained kidney beans
1 cup vegetable broth
1 cup cooked quinoa
1 teaspoon ground cumin
1/2 teaspoon chili powder
1/4 teaspoon smoked paprika
Salt and pepper to taste
Optional toppings: Chopped avocado, shredded cheese, low-fat Greek yogurt, chopped fresh cilantro

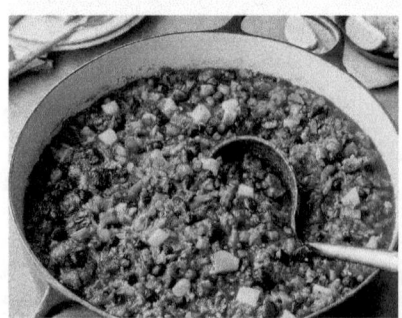

Vegetarian Chili with Quinoa and Black Beans

4 servings 45 minutes

DIRECTIONS

- In a big pot or Dutch oven, warm up the olive oil over medium heat.
- Add onion, garlic, bell pepper, and jalapeño (if using). Simmer for five minutes, or until tender.
- Stir in diced tomatoes, black beans, kidney beans, vegetable broth, cooked quinoa, cumin, chili powder, smoked paprika, salt, and pepper.
- Bring to a boil, then reduce heat and simmer for 20-25 minutes, or until flavors meld and chili thickens slightly.
- Serve hot with your favorite toppings (optional).

NUTRITIONAL VALUE (APPROXIMATE)

- Calories: 400
- Protein: 20g
- Fat: 10g (healthy fats from olive oil)
- Carbs: 50g (fiber: 10g)

Lentil and Vegetable Soup with Whole-Wheat Bread

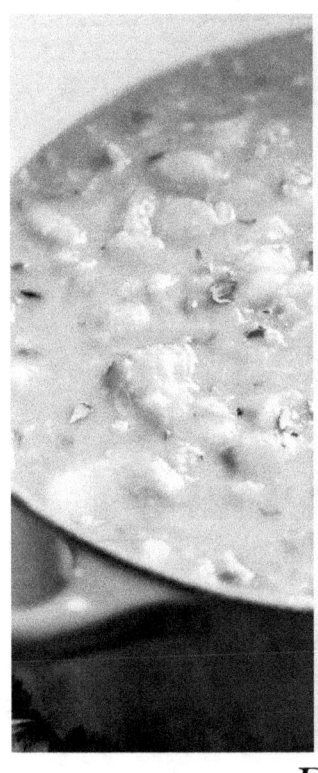

 4 servings   45 minutes

INGREDIENTS

1 tablespoon olive oil
1 onion, chopped
2 cloves garlic, minced
1 carrot, chopped
1 celery stalk, chopped
1 cup brown lentils, rinsed
4 cups vegetable broth
1 (14.5 oz) can diced tomatoes, undrained
1 teaspoon dried thyme
1/2 teaspoon dried oregano
Salt and pepper to taste
Whole-wheat bread slices (for serving)

DIRECTIONS

- In a big pot or Dutch oven over medium heat, warm the olive oil.
- Add onion, garlic, carrot, and celery. Simmer for five minutes, or until tender.
- Add lentils, vegetable broth, diced tomatoes, thyme, oregano, salt, and pepper.
- Bring to a boil, then reduce heat and simmer for 30 minutes, or until lentils are tender.
- Serve hot with slices of whole-wheat bread.

NUTRITIONAL VALUE (APPROXIMATE):

- Calories: 350
- Protein: 15g
- Fat: 5g (healthy fats from olive oil)
- Carbs: 50g (fiber: 10g)

Snacks

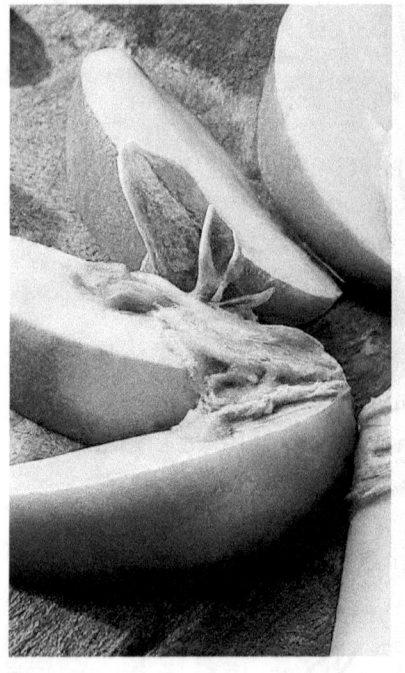

Apple Slices with Almond Butter

🍴 1 serving   🕐 2 minutes

INGREDIENTS

1 apple, sliced
2 tablespoons almond butter

DIRECTIONS

- Wash and slice the apple.
- Spread almond butter on the apple slices.

NUTRITIONAL VALUE (APPROXIMATE):

- Calories: 200
- Protein: 5g
- Fat: 10g (healthy fats from almond butter)
- Carbs: 25g (fiber: 3g)

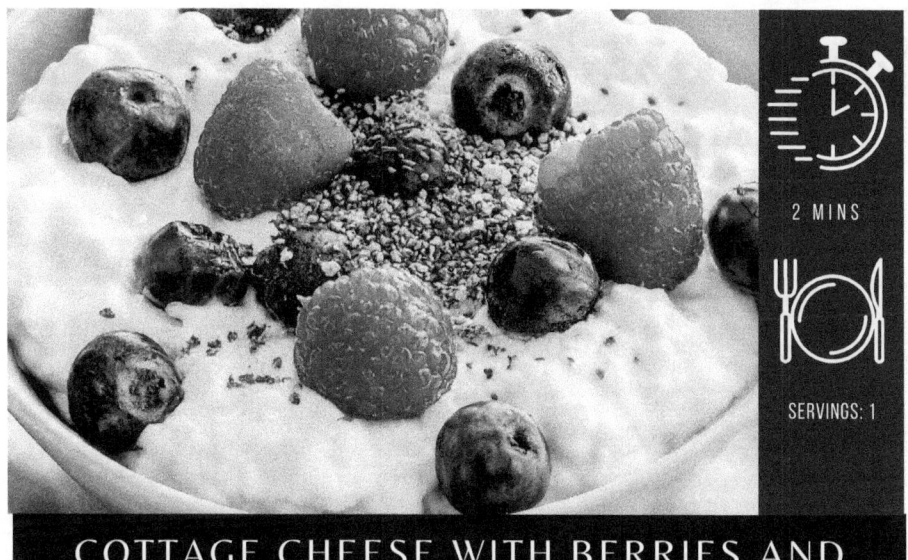

2 MINS

SERVINGS: 1

COTTAGE CHEESE WITH BERRIES AND CHIA SEEDS

INGREDIENTS

- 1/2 cup low-fat cottage cheese
- 1/4 cup mixed berries
- 1 tablespoon chia seeds

DIRECTIONS

1. Combine cottage cheese, berries, and chia seeds in a bowl.

NUTRITIONAL VALUE(APPROXIMATE):

- Calories: 150
- Protein: 12g
- Fat: 3g
- Carbs: 15g (fiber: 3g)

Edamame Pods with Sea Salt

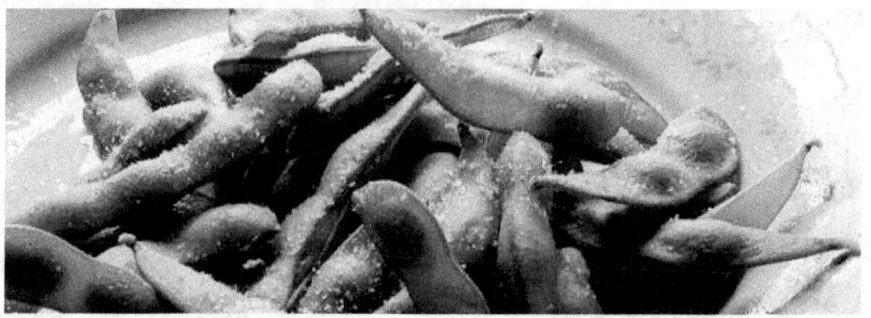

Ingredients:

- 1 cup frozen edamame pods, thawed
- Pinch of sea salt

Instructions:

- Thaw frozen edamame pods according to package instructions.
- Sprinkle with a pinch of sea salt.

Nutritional Value (Approximate):

- Calories: 150
- Protein: 17g
- Fat: 5g (healthy fats)
- Carbs: 10g (fiber: 2g)

Servings: 1

Preparation time : 2 mins

Roasted Chickpeas with Spices

INGREDIENTS

1 cup canned chickpeas, rinsed and drained
1 tablespoon olive oil
1/2 teaspoon ground cumin
1/4 teaspoon paprika
Salt and pepper to taste

 1 serving   25 minutes

DIRECTIONS

1. Preheat oven to 400°F (200°C).
2. Toss chickpeas with olive oil, cumin, paprika, salt, and pepper.
3. On a baking sheet, distribute the chickpeas in a single layer.
4. Roast for 20-25 minutes, or until golden brown and crispy.

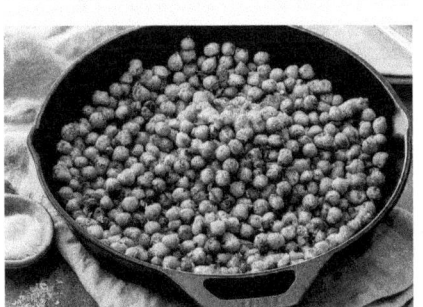

NUTRITIONAL VALUE (APPROXIMATE)

Calories: 300
Protein: 8g
Fat: 10g (healthy fats from flaxseed)
Carbs: 35g (fiber: 5g)

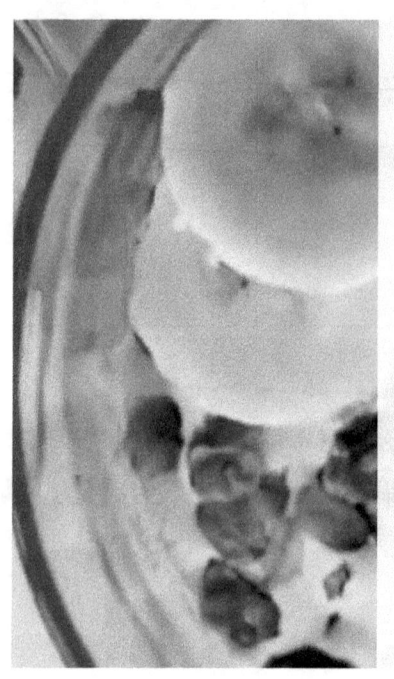

Greek Yogurt with Sliced Banana and Walnuts

 1 serving   2 minutes

INGREDIENTS

1/2 cup plain Greek yogurt (2% fat)
1/2 banana, sliced
1/4 cup chopped walnuts

DIRECTIONS

- In a bowl, combine Greek yogurt, sliced banana, and chopped walnuts.

NUTRITIONAL VALUE (APPROXIMATE):

- Calories: 250
- Protein: 15g
- Fat: 10g (healthy fats from walnuts)
- Carbs: 25g (fiber: 3g)

Salads

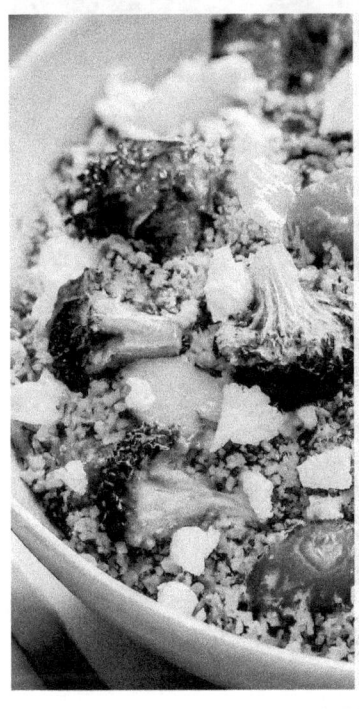

Quinoa Salad with Roasted Vegetables and Feta

🍴 2 servings   25 minutes

INGREDIENTS

1 cup cooked quinoa
1 cup assorted vegetables
(broccoli florets, cherry tomatoes, bell pepper chunks)
1 tablespoon olive oil
1/4 cup crumbled feta cheese
2 tablespoons lemon juice
1 tablespoon olive oil (for dressing)
1/2 teaspoon dried oregano
Salt and pepper to taste

DIRECTIONS

- Preheat the oven to 400°F (200°C).
- Combine one tablespoon of olive oil, salt, and pepper with the vegetables.
- Spread the vegetables on a baking sheet and roast for 15 minutes, or until tender-crisp.
- While the vegetables roast, whisk together lemon juice, 1 tablespoon olive oil, and oregano for the dressing.
- In a bowl, combine cooked quinoa, roasted vegetables, crumbled feta cheese, and dressing.
- After tossing to coat, add more salt and pepper to taste.

NUTRITIONAL VALUE (APPROXIMATE):

- Calories: 400
- Protein: 15g
- Fat: 15g (healthy fats from olive oil and feta)
- Carbs: 40g (fiber: 5g)

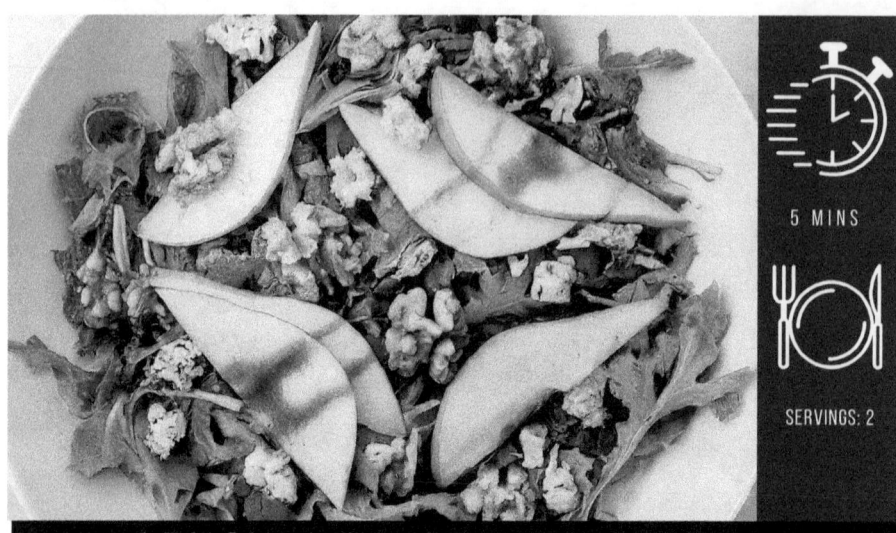

5 MINS

SERVINGS: 2

ARUGULA SALAD WITH PEARS, WALNUTS, AND BLUE CHEESE

INGREDIENTS

- 4 cups baby arugula
- 1 ripe pear, thinly sliced
- 1/4 cup chopped walnuts
- 2 ounces crumbled blue cheese
- 2 tablespoons balsamic vinegar
- 1 tablespoon olive oil
- Salt and pepper to taste

DIRECTIONS

- In a large bowl, combine baby arugula, sliced pears, chopped walnuts, and crumbled blue cheese.
- In a small bowl, whisk together balsamic vinegar and olive oil for the dressing.
- After adding the salad dressing, toss to coat.
- Season with salt and pepper to taste.

NUTRITIONAL VALUE(APPROXIMATE):

- Calories: 450
- Protein: 10g
- Fat: 25g (healthy fats from walnuts and blue cheese)
- Carbs: 35g (fiber: 4g)

Lentil Salad with Cucumber, Tomato, and Lemon Dill Dressing

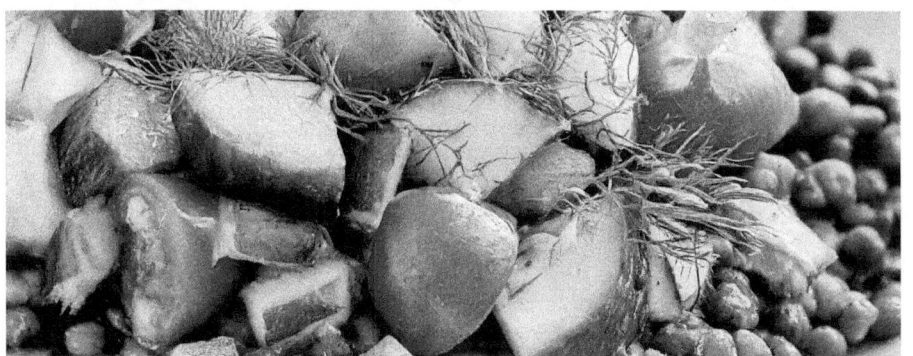

Ingredients:

- 1 cup cooked lentils
- 1 cucumber, diced
- 1 tomato, diced
- 1/4 cup chopped red onion
- 1/4 cup chopped fresh dill
- 2 tablespoons lemon juice
- 1 tablespoon olive oil
- Salt and pepper to taste

Instructions:

- In a large bowl, combine cooked lentils, diced cucumber, tomato, and red onion.
- In a small bowl, whisk together lemon juice, olive oil, and chopped dill for the dressing.
- After adding the dressing, toss the salad to coat.
- Season with salt and pepper to taste.

Nutritional Value (Approximate):

- Calories: 300
- Protein: 18g
- Fat: 5g (healthy fats from olive oil)
- Carbs: 40g (fiber: 10g)

Servings: 2   Preparation time : 15 mins

Greek Salad with Grilled Chicken and Lemon Oregano Vinaigrette

INGREDIENTS

1. 4 cups mixed greens
2. 1 boneless, skinless chicken breast, grilled or cooked
3. 1/2 cup crumbled feta cheese
4. 1/4 cup sliced Kalamata olives
5. 1 red onion, thinly sliced
6. 2 tablespoons olive oil
7. 1 tablespoon lemon juice
8. 1/2 teaspoon dried oregano
9. Salt and pepper to taste

 2 serving   20 minutes

DIRECTIONS

1. Grill or cook the chicken breast and slice it into strips.
2. In a large bowl, combine mixed greens, sliced chicken strips, crumbled feta cheese, Kalamata olives, and red onion slices
3. Preparation (Continued): 3. In a small bowl, whisk together olive oil, lemon juice, oregano, salt, and pepper for the dressing.
4. Toss to coat the salad after drizzling with dressing.
5. Season with additional salt and pepper to taste.

NUTRITIONAL VALUE (APPROXIMATE)
- Calories: 450
- Protein: 35g
- Fat: 20g (healthy fats from olive oil and feta cheese)
- Carbs: 20g (fiber: 3g)

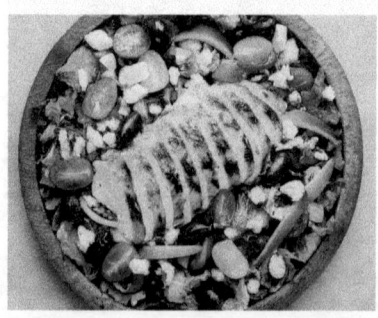

Tuna Salad with Celery, Grapes, and Walnuts

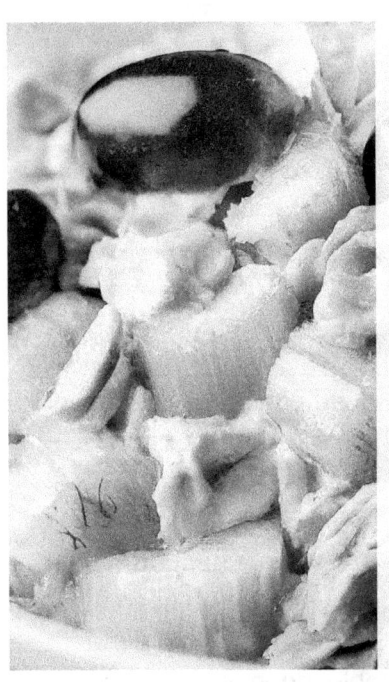

2 servings · 10 minutes

INGREDIENTS

Two drained cans (5 oz each) of tuna in water
1/2 cup chopped celery
1/4 cup red grapes, halved
1/4 cup chopped walnuts
2 tablespoons plain Greek yogurt (2% fat)
1 tablespoon lemon juice
1/2 teaspoon dried dill
Salt and pepper to taste

DIRECTIONS

- In a large bowl, combine drained tuna, chopped celery, halved grapes, and chopped walnuts.
- In a small bowl, whisk together Greek yogurt, lemon juice, dill, salt, and pepper for the dressing.
- After adding the dressing, toss the salad to coat.
- Season with additional salt and pepper to taste.

NUTRITIONAL VALUE (APPROXIMATE):

- Calories: 400
- Protein: 30g
- Fat: 15g (healthy fats from walnuts)
- Carbs: 25g (fiber: 2g)

Soups

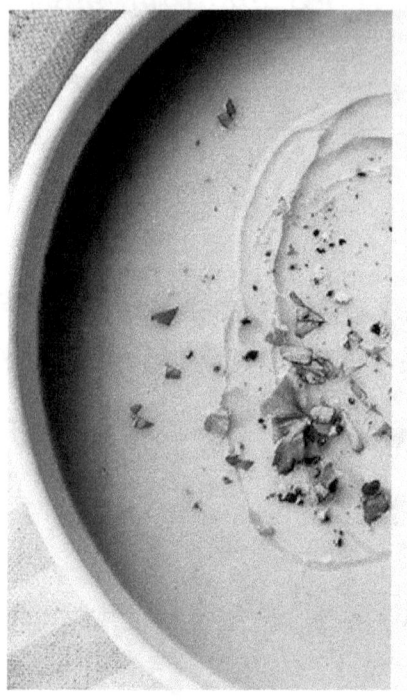

Lentil Soup with Lemon and Herbs

2 servings 30 minutes

INGREDIENTS

1 cup dried brown lentils, rinsed
4 cups vegetable broth
1 carrot, chopped
1 celery stalk, chopped
1/2 onion, chopped
1 clove garlic, minced
1 tablespoon olive oil
1 tablespoon lemon juice
1/4 cup chopped fresh herbs
(parsley, dill, or thyme)
Salt and pepper to taste

DIRECTIONS

- Olive oil should be heated over medium heat in a big pot.
- Add chopped onion and celery, and cook for 5 minutes, or until softened.
- Add chopped carrot and garlic, cook for an additional minute.
- Add rinsed lentils and vegetable broth to the pot.
- Bring to a boil, then reduce heat and simmer for 20 minutes, or until lentils are tender.
- Stir in lemon juice and chopped herbs.
- Season with salt and pepper to taste.

NUTRITIONAL VALUE (APPROXIMATE):

- Calories: 300
- Protein: 18g
- Fat: 5g (healthy fats from olive oil)
- Carbs: 40g (fiber: 10g)

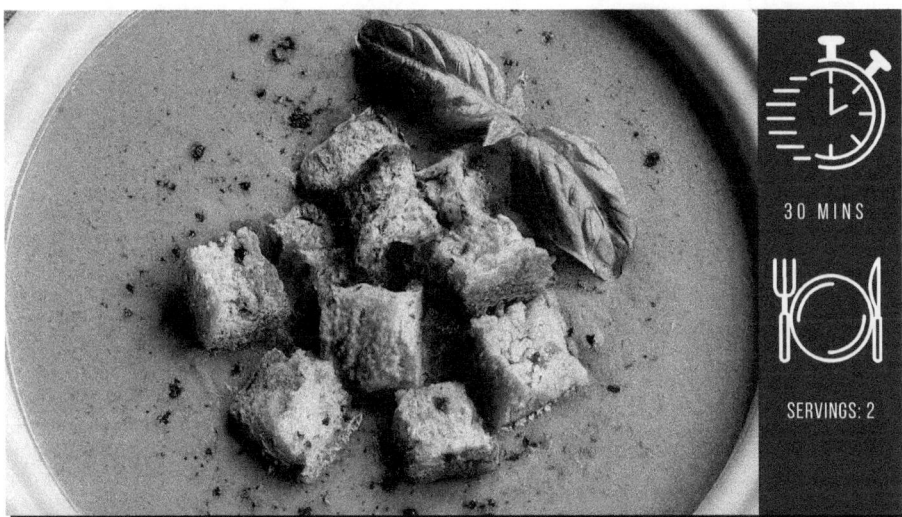

30 MINS

SERVINGS: 2

TOMATO AND BASIL SOUP WITH WHOLE WHEAT CROUTONS

INGREDIENTS

- 1 (28-ounce) can crushed tomatoes
- 1 cup vegetable broth
- 1/2 onion, chopped
- 2 cloves garlic, minced
- 1 tablespoon olive oil
- 1/4 cup chopped fresh basil
- Two slices of diced and toasted whole wheat bread
- Salt and pepper to taste

NUTRITIONAL VALUE(APPROXIMATE):
- Calories: 250
- Protein: 5g
- Fat: 5g
- Carbs: 40g (fiber: 5g)

DIRECTIONS

- Pour olive oil into a big pot and warm it up on medium heat
- Add chopped onion and garlic, cook for 5 minutes, or until softened.
- Add crushed tomatoes and vegetable broth to the pot.
- Bring to a boil, then simmer for fifteen minutes on low heat.
- Stir in chopped fresh basil.
- Using an immersion blender or food processor, puree the soup until desired consistency is reached.
- Season with salt and pepper to taste.
- Serve with toasted whole wheat bread cubes.

Chicken Noodle Soup with Vegetables

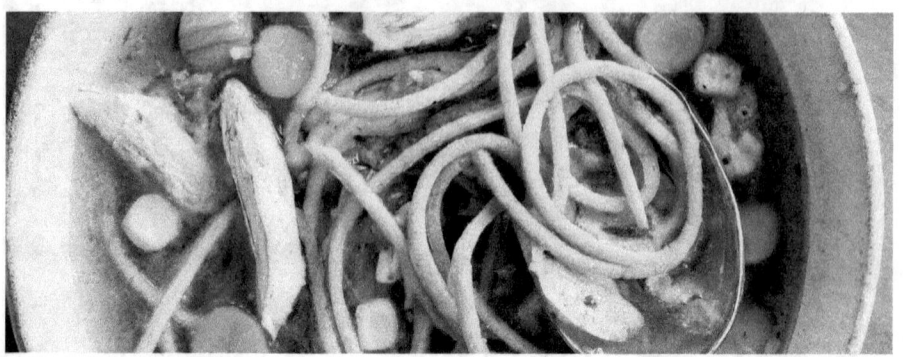

Ingredients:

- One cooked and shredded boneless, skinless chicken breast
- 4 cups chicken broth (low-sodium preferred)
- 1 cup chopped vegetables (carrots, celery, peas)
- 1/2 onion, chopped
- 1 clove garlic, minced
- 1 tablespoon olive oil
- 1/2 cup cooked whole wheat noodles
- Salt and pepper to taste

Instructions:

- Warm up the olive oil in a large skillet over medium heat.
- Add chopped onion and garlic, cook for 5 minutes, or until softened.
- Add chopped vegetables and chicken broth to the pot.
- The veggies should be soft after ten minutes of simmering at a reduced heat after bringing to a boil.
- Add cooked shredded chicken and cooked whole wheat noodles to the pot.
- Heat through for an additional 5 minutes.
- Season with salt and pepper to taste.

Nutritional Value (Approximate):

Calories: 250
Protein: 12g
Fat: 15g
Carbs: 5g (fiber: 2g)

Servings: 2   Preparation time : 30 mins

Curried Butternut Squash Soup with Coconut Milk

★★★★☆

 2 serving    30 minutes

INGREDIENTS

- 1 medium butternut squash, peeled and cubed
- 1 cup vegetable broth
- 1/2 cup light coconut milk
- 1 tablespoon curry powder
- 1 teaspoon ground ginger
- 1/2 onion, chopped
- 1 clove garlic, minced
- 1 tablespoon olive oil
- Salt and pepper to taste

DIRECTIONS

- Olive oil should be heated over medium heat in a big pot.
- Add chopped onion and garlic, cook for 3 minutes, or until softened.
- Add curry powder and ginger, cook for an additional minute, stirring constantly.
- Add cubed butternut squash and vegetable broth to the pot.
- Bring to a boil, then reduce heat and simmer for 15 minutes, or until the squash is tender.
- Stir in light coconut milk and heat through.
- Using an immersion blender or food processor, puree the soup until desired consistency is reached.
- Season with salt and pepper to taste.

NUTRITIONAL VALUE (APPROXIMATE)

- Calories: 350
- Protein: 4g
- Fat: 18g
- Carbs: 30g (fiber: 5g)

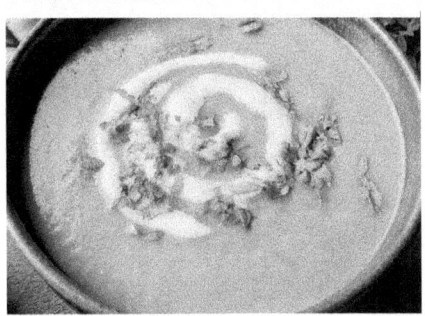

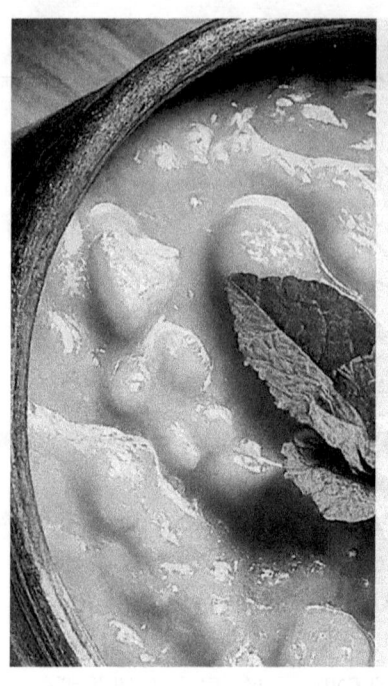

Split Pea Soup with Lemon and Mint

 2 servings   30 minutes

INGREDIENTS

1 cup dried green split peas, rinsed
4 cups vegetable broth
1 carrot, chopped
1 celery stalk, chopped
1/2 onion, chopped
1 tablespoon olive oil
1 tablespoon lemon juice
1 tablespoon chopped fresh mint
Salt and pepper to taste

DIRECTIONS

- Begin to warm up the olive oil in a big pot over medium heat.
- Add chopped onion, celery, and carrot, cook for 5 minutes, or until softened.
- Add rinsed split peas and vegetable broth to the pot.
- Bring to a boil, then reduce heat and simmer for 20 minutes, or until split peas are tender.
- Stir in lemon juice and chopped fresh mint.
- Using an immersion blender or food processor, puree the soup until desired consistency is reached.
- Season with salt and pepper to taste.

NUTRITIONAL VALUE (APPROXIMATE):

- Calories: 250
- Protein: 15g
- Fat: 5g (healthy fats from olive oil)
- Carbs: 40g (fiber: 10g)

Stews

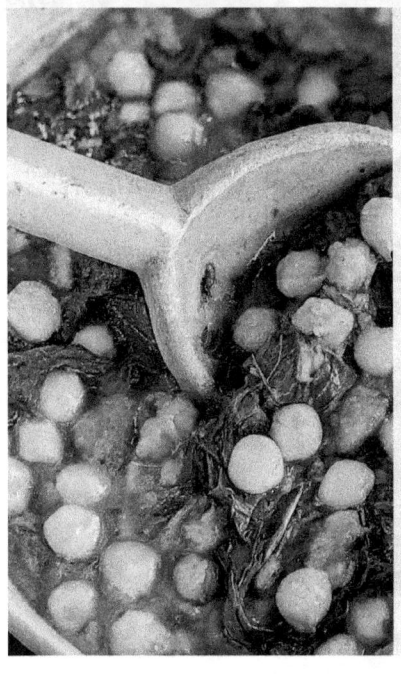

Mediterranean Chickpea Stew with Tomatoes and Spinach

 2 servings   40 minutes

INGREDIENTS

1 (15-ounce) can chickpeas, rinsed and drained
1 (14.5-ounce) can diced tomatoes, undrained
1 cup vegetable broth
1/2 cup chopped red onion
2 cloves garlic, minced
1 tablespoon olive oil
1/2 teaspoon dried oregano
1/4 teaspoon dried thyme
1 cup chopped fresh spinach
Salt and pepper to taste

DIRECTIONS

- Olive oil should be heated over medium heat in a big pot.
- Add chopped onion and garlic, cook for 5 minutes, or until softened.
- Add diced tomatoes (with juices), vegetable broth, oregano, and thyme to the pot.
- After bringing to a boil, lower the heat, and simmer for approximately fifteen minutes.
- Stir in rinsed and drained chickpeas and chopped fresh spinach.
- Cook for an additional 5 minutes, or until spinach is wilted.
- Season with salt and pepper to taste.

NUTRITIONAL VALUE (APPROXIMATE):

- Calories: 300
- Protein: 15g
- Fat: 5g (healthy fats from olive oil)
- Carbs: 40g (fiber: 10g)

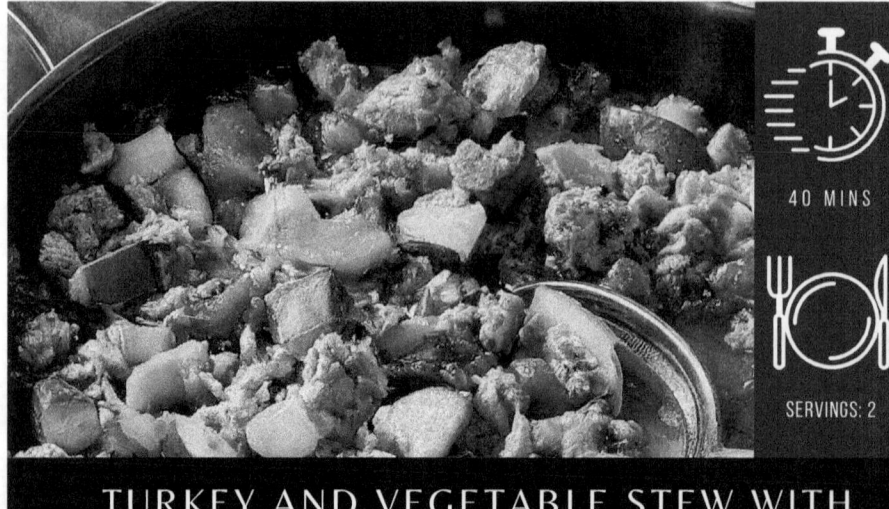

40 MINS

SERVINGS: 2

TURKEY AND VEGETABLE STEW WITH BROWN RICE

INGREDIENTS

- 1 pound ground turkey
- 1 cup chopped vegetables (carrots, celery, zucchini)
- 1/2 cup chopped onion
- 2 cloves garlic, minced
- 1 tablespoon olive oil
- 1 (14.5-ounce) can diced tomatoes, undrained
- 1 cup low-sodium chicken broth
- 1/2 cup cooked brown rice
- Salt and pepper to taste

DIRECTIONS

1. Olive oil should be warmed over medium heat in a big pot.
2. Add chopped onion and garlic, cook for 5 minutes, or until softened.
3. Using a spoon, break up the ground turkey and sauté it until it turns brown.
4. Add chopped vegetables, diced tomatoes (with juices), and chicken broth to the pot.
5. The veggies should be soft after 20 minutes of cooking at a reduced heat after bringing to a boil.
6. Stir in cooked brown rice and heat through for an additional 5 minutes.
7. Season with salt and pepper to taste.

NUTRITIONAL VALUE(APPROXIMATE):

- Calories: 400
- Protein: 35g
- Fat: 10g (healthy fats from olive oil)
- Carbs: 35g (fiber: 5g)

Beef and Butternut Squash Stew with Whole Wheat Couscous

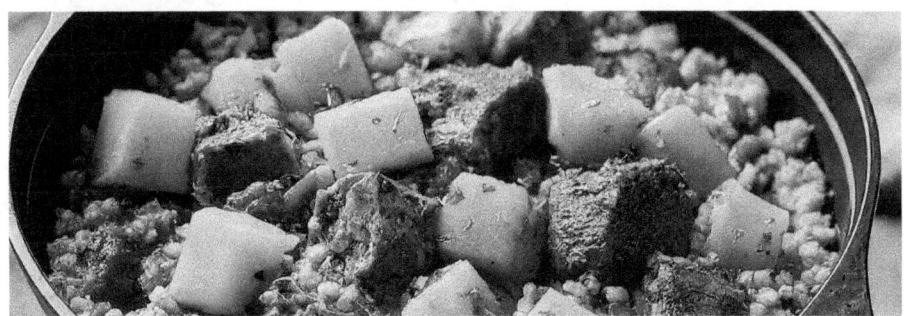

Ingredients:

- 1 pound lean beef stew meat, trimmed and cut into bite-sized pieces
- 1 medium butternut squash, peeled and cubed
- 1 cup chopped vegetables (carrots, celery)
- 1/2 cup chopped onion
- 2 cloves garlic, minced
- 1 tablespoon olive oil
- 4 cups low-sodium beef broth
- 1/2 cup cooked whole wheat couscous
- Salt and pepper to taste

Nutritional Value (Approximate):

- Calories: 500
- Protein: 40g
- Fat: 15g (healthy fats from olive oil)
- Carbs: 40g (fiber: 5g)

Servings: 2

Instructions:

- Olive oil should be heated over medium-high heat in a big pot or Dutch oven.
- Sear the beef stew meat on all sides until browned.
- Remove the beef and set aside.
- Add chopped onion and garlic to the pot, cook for 5 minutes, or until softened.
- Add chopped vegetables and cubed butternut squash to the pot.
- Cook for an additional 5 minutes, or until vegetables start to soften.
- Add low-sodium beef broth and bring to a boil.
- Reduce heat, return the browned beef to the pot, and simmer for 20 minutes, or until the beef and vegetables are tender.
- Stir in cooked whole wheat couscous and heat through for an additional 5 minutes.
- Season with salt and pepper to taste.

Preparation time : 45 mins

Lentil and Mushroom Stew with Barley

INGREDIENTS

 2 servings   40 minutes

DIRECTIONS

1 cup dried brown lentils, rinsed
1 cup sliced mushrooms
1/2 cup chopped onion
2 cloves garlic, minced
1 tablespoon olive oil
4 cups vegetable broth
1/2 cup cooked barley
1 tablespoon chopped fresh parsley
Salt and pepper to taste

- Pour olive oil into a big pot and then heat it up on medium heat.
- Add chopped onion and garlic, cook for 5 minutes, or until softened.
- Add sliced mushrooms and cook for an additional 5 minutes, or until browned.
- Add rinsed lentils and vegetable broth to the pot.
- Bring to a boil, then reduce heat and simmer for 20 minutes, or until lentils are tender.
- Stir in cooked barley and chopped fresh parsley.
- Cook for an additional 5 minutes.
- Season with salt and pepper to taste.

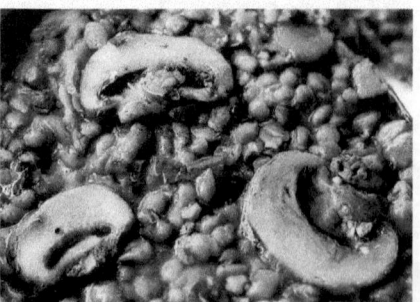

NUTRITIONAL VALUE (APPROXIMATE)

- Calories: 350
- Protein: 20g
- Fat: 5g (healthy fats from olive oil)
- Carbs: 50g (fiber: 15g)

Chicken and White Bean Stew with Kale

2 servings — 40 minutes

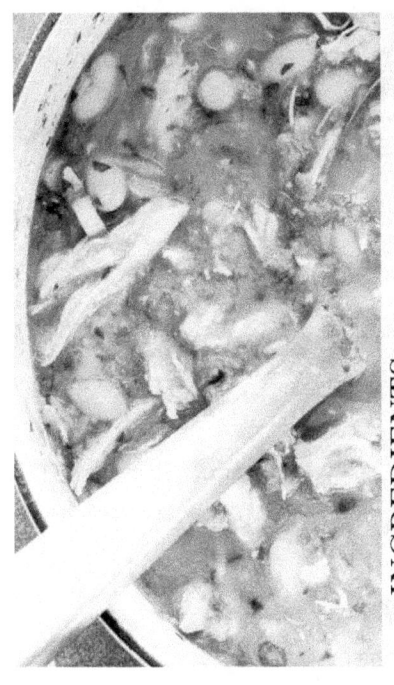

INGREDIENTS

- One cooked, shredded, skinless, and boneless chicken breast
- One fifteen-ounce can of rinsed and drained cannellini beans
- 1 cup chopped vegetables (carrots, celery)
- 1/2 cup chopped onion
- 2 cloves garlic, minced
- 1 tablespoon olive oil
- 4 cups vegetable broth
- 2 cups chopped kale, ribs removed
- Salt and pepper to taste

DIRECTIONS

- In a large saucepan, the olive oil should be heated over medium heat.
- Add chopped onion and garlic, cook for 5 minutes, or until softened.
- Add chopped vegetables and cook for an additional 5 minutes, or until vegetables start to soften.
- Bring the vegetable broth to a boil after adding it.
- Reduce heat, simmer for 10 minutes.
- Stir in rinsed and drained cannellini beans and cooked shredded chicken.
- Cook for an additional 5 minutes.
- Add chopped kale and cook for another 2-3 minutes, or until kale is wilted.
- Season with salt and pepper to taste.

NUTRITIONAL VALUE (APPROXIMATE):

- Calories: 400
- Protein: 30g
- Fat: 5g (healthy fats from olive oil)
- Carbs: 50g (fiber: 10g)

Fish Recipes

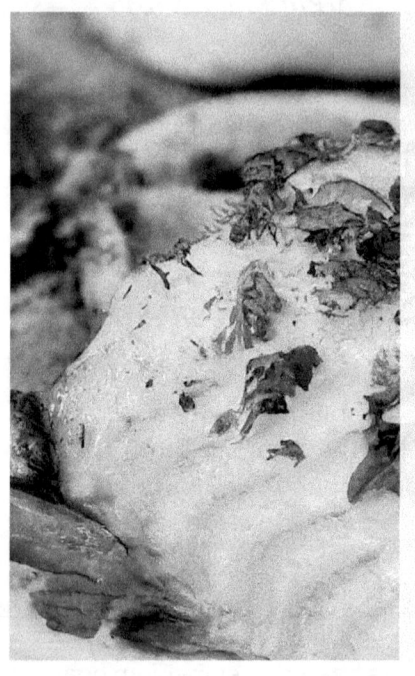

Baked Cod with Lemon and Herbs

2 servings   30 minutes

INGREDIENTS

2 cod filets (around 4-6 oz each)
1 tablespoon olive oil
1/2 lemon, sliced
1 tablespoon chopped fresh parsley
1/2 teaspoon dried thyme
Salt and pepper to taste

DIRECTIONS

- Preheat the oven to 400°F (200°C).
- Lightly grease a baking dish.
- Cod filets should be placed in the prepared baking dish.
- Season with salt and pepper and sprinkle with olive oil.
- Top with lemon slices, chopped parsley, and dried thyme.
- Fish should flake readily with a fork after 20 minutes of baking.

NUTRITIONAL VALUE (APPROXIMATE):

- Calories: 300
- Protein: 35g
- Fat: 10g (healthy fats from olive oil)
- Carbs: 5g

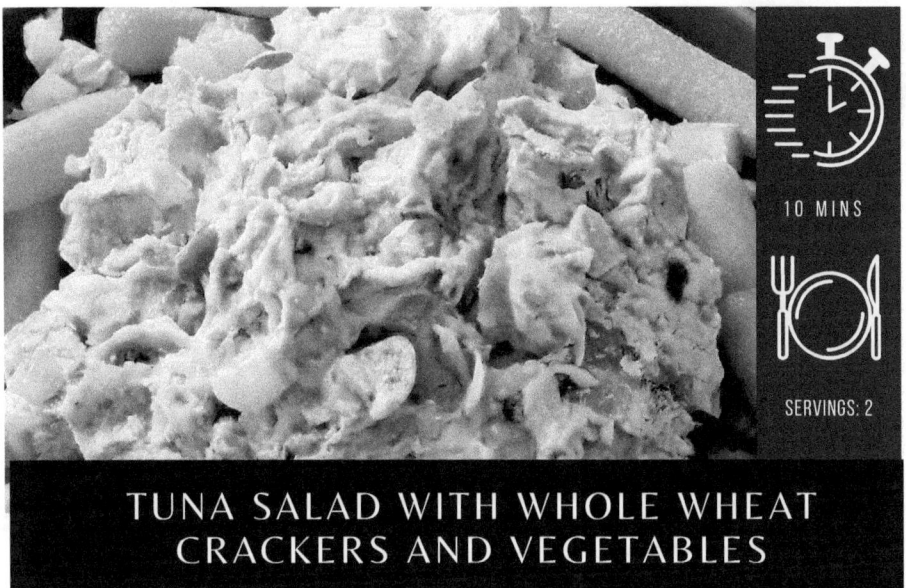

TUNA SALAD WITH WHOLE WHEAT CRACKERS AND VEGETABLES

INGREDIENTS

- 2 cans (5 oz each) tuna in water(water-packed tuna), drained
- 1/4 cup chopped celery
- 1/4 cup chopped red onion
- 2 tablespoons plain Greek yogurt (2% fat)
- 1 tablespoon lemon juice
- 1/2 teaspoon dried dill
- Salt and pepper to taste
- Whole wheat crackers and baby carrots (for serving)

DIRECTIONS

1. In a large bowl, combine drained tuna, chopped celery, and chopped red onion.
2. In a small bowl, whisk together Greek yogurt, lemon juice, dill, salt, and pepper for the dressing.
3. After pouring the dressing over the salad, mix to coat.
4. Serve with whole wheat crackers and baby carrots for a complete meal.

NUTRITIONAL VALUE(APPROXIMATE):

- Calories: 350
- Protein: 30g
- Fat: 5g (healthy fats from yogurt)
- Carbs: 30g (fiber: 3g)

CONSUME THIS RECIPE IN MODERATION

Pan-Seared Salmon with Garlic and Spinach

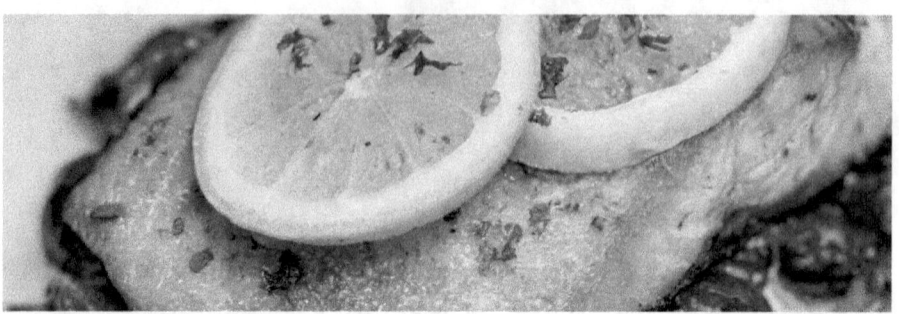

Ingredients:

- 2 salmon fillets (around 4-6 oz each)
- 1 tablespoon olive oil
- 2 cloves garlic, minced
- 4 cups baby spinach
- 1/4 cup low-sodium chicken broth
- 1 tablespoon lemon juice
- Salt and pepper to taste

Instructions:

- In a large pan, preheat the olive oil over medium heat.
- Season salmon filets with salt and pepper.
- Salmon filets should be seared for 3–4 minutes on each side, or until done.
- Take out and place aside the salmon from the pan.
- Add minced garlic to the pan and cook for 30 seconds, until fragrant.
- Add baby spinach and cook until wilted.
- Pour in chicken broth and lemon juice, scraping any browned bits from the bottom of the pan.
- Season with additional salt and pepper to taste.
- Plate the salmon fillets and spoon the spinach mixture over the top.

Nutritional Value (Approximate):

- Calories: 400
- Protein: 40g
- Fat: 15g (healthy fats from salmon)
- Carbs: 5g (fiber: 2g)

Servings: 2 *Preparation time : 25 mins*

Poached Tilapia with Vegetables and Dill Sauce

 2 servings   25 minutes

INGREDIENTS

- 2 tilapia fillets (around 4-6 oz each)
- 2 cups vegetable broth
- 1 cup chopped vegetables (carrots, celery)
- 1/2 lemon, sliced
- 1/4 cup chopped fresh dill
- 1 tablespoon low-fat yogurt
- Salt and pepper to taste

DIRECTIONS

- In a large pot, combine vegetable broth, chopped vegetables, and lemon slices.
- bring to a boil, then cook for five minutes on low heat.
- Gently place tilapia filets in the simmering broth.
- Fish should flake readily with a fork after 10 to 12 minutes of cooking while covered.
- While the fish cooks, combine chopped dill and low-fat yogurt in a small bowl.
- Plate the fish and vegetables, spooning the dill sauce over the top.

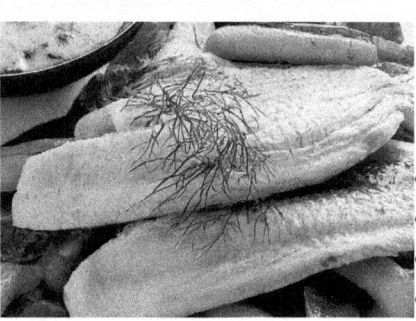

NUTRITIONAL VALUE (APPROXIMATE)

- Calories: 250
- Protein: 30g
- Fat: 5g (healthy fats from yogurt)
- Carbs: 10g (fiber: 2g)

Baked Haddock with Tomato and Herbs

2 servings | 30 minutes

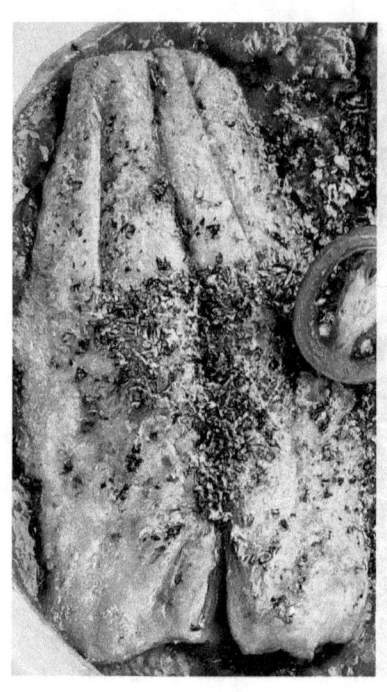

INGREDIENTS

2 haddock filets (around 4-6 oz each)
1 tablespoon olive oil
1 (14.5-ounce) can diced tomatoes, undrained
1/4 cup chopped fresh basil
1/4 cup chopped fresh oregano
1/4 cup chopped red onion
Salt and pepper to taste

DIRECTIONS

- Preheat the oven to 400°F (200°C).
- Lightly grease a baking dish.
- Place haddock filets in the prepared baking dish.
- Drizzle with olive oil before garnishing with salt and pepper.
- In a small bowl, combine diced tomatoes (with juices), chopped basil, chopped oregano, and chopped red onion.
- Spoon the tomato mixture over the haddock filets.
- Bake for 20 minutes, or until the fish flakes easily with a fork and the tomato mixture is bubbly.

NUTRITIONAL VALUE (APPROXIMATE):

- Calories: 350
- Protein: 30g
- Fat: 10g (healthy fats from olive oil)
- Carbs: 20g (fiber: 2g)

Dessert

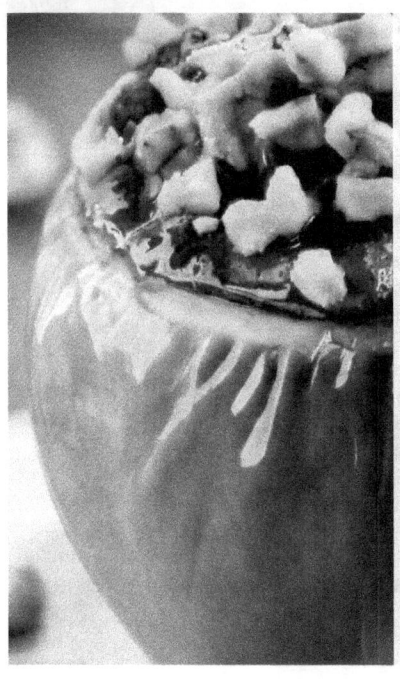

Baked Apples with Cinnamon and Walnuts

 1 serving   25 minutes

INGREDIENTS

- 1 apple, cored
- 1/4 cup chopped walnuts
- 1 tablespoon honey
- 1/2 teaspoon ground cinnamon
- Pinch of nutmeg (optional)

DIRECTIONS

- Preheat oven to 375°F (190°C).
- In a small bowl, combine chopped walnuts, honey, cinnamon, and nutmeg (optional).
- Stuff the apple core with the walnut mixture.
- Place the apple in a baking dish and bake for 15 minutes, or until tender.

NUTRITIONAL VALUE (APPROXIMATE):
- Calories: 250
- Protein: 2g
- Fat: 10g (healthy fats from walnuts)
- Carbs: 35g (fiber: 4g)

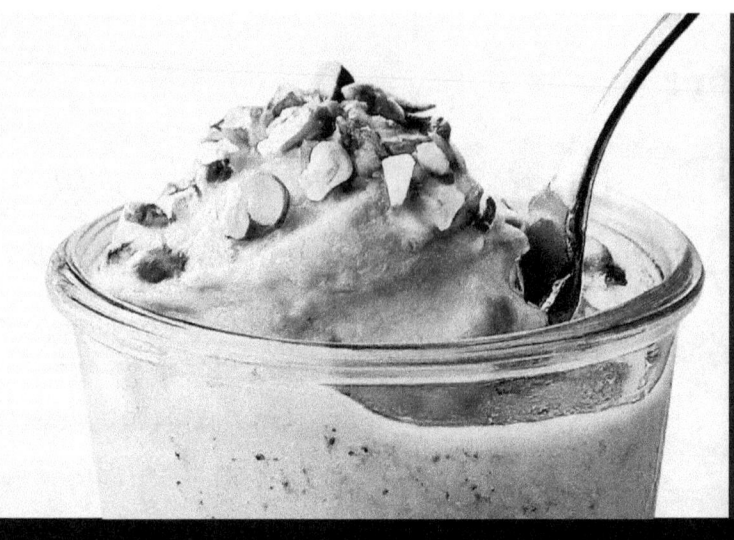
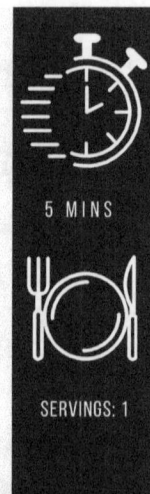

5 MINS

SERVINGS: 1

FROZEN BANANA "NICE CREAM"

INGREDIENTS

- 1 ripe banana, frozen and sliced
- One-fourth cup of almond milk, unsweetened (or your preferred milk)
- 1/2 teaspoon vanilla extract (optional)
- Optional toppings: Chopped nuts, cocoa powder, berries

DIRECTIONS

- Freeze ripe banana slices for at least 2-4 hours, or until frozen solid.
- Blend frozen banana slices, almond milk, and vanilla extract (optional) in a blender or food processor until smooth and creamy.
- Serve immediately topped with your favorite ingredients (optional).

NUTRITIONAL VALUE(APPROXIMATE):

- Calories: 200
- Protein: 1g
- Fat: 5g (healthy fats)
- Carbs: 30g (fiber: 2g)

Baked Pears with Ginger and Spices

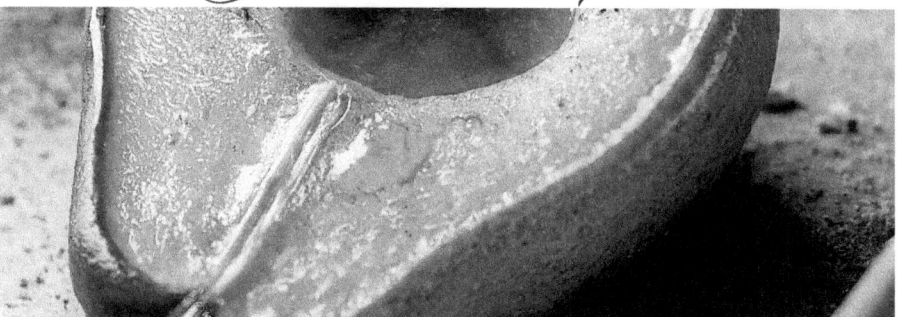

Ingredients:

- 1 pear, halved and cored
- 1 tablespoon honey
- 1/2 teaspoon ground ginger
- 1/4 teaspoon ground cloves
- Pinch of nutmeg

Instructions:

1. Preheat the oven to 375°F (190°C).
2. In a small bowl, combine honey, ginger, cloves, and nutmeg.
3. Brush the pear halves with the honey mixture.
4. Place the pear halves in a baking dish, cut side down.
5. Bake for 15 minutes, or until tender and slightly softened.

Nutritional Value (Approximate):

- Calories: 200
- Protein: 0g
- Fat: 0g
- Carbs: 50g (fiber: 5g)

Servings: 1   Preparation time : 25 mins

Greek Yogurt Parfait with Berries and Granola

INGREDIENTS

 1 serving 5 minutes

1/2 cup plain Greek yogurt (2% fat)
1/4 cup mixed berries
1/4 cup granola (choose a low-sugar option)

DIRECTIONS

In a bowl, layer Greek yogurt, mixed berries, and granola.

NUTRITIONAL VALUE (APPROXIMATE)

- Calories: 250
- Protein: 15g
- Fat: 5g (healthy fats)
- Carbs: 30g (fiber: 3g)

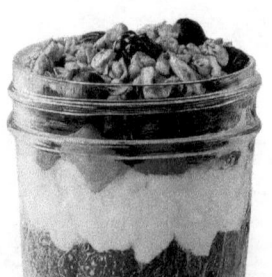

Dates with Nut Butter and Dark Chocolate

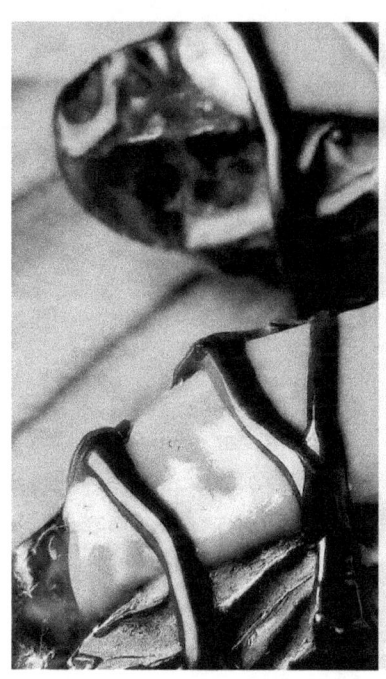

 1 serving   2 minutes

INGREDIENTS

- 2 Medjool dates
- 1 tablespoon of nut butter, for instance almond butter
- 1 square dark chocolate (at least 70% cacao)

DIRECTIONS

- Pit the dates.
- Stuff each date with a spoonful of nut butter.
- Top with a small square of dark chocolate.

NUTRITIONAL VALUE (APPROXIMATE):

- Calories: 200
- Protein: 2g
- Fat: 10g (healthy fats from nut butter and dark chocolate)
- Carbs: 30g (fiber: 4g)

Vegetable Recipes

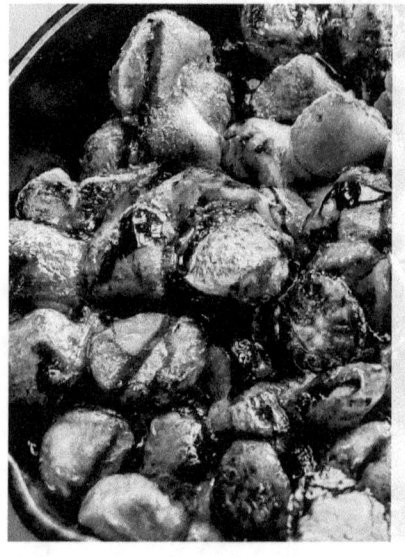

Roasted Brussels Sprouts with Balsamic Glaze

2 servings   30 minutes

INGREDIENTS

1 pound Brussels sprouts, trimmed and halved
1 tablespoon olive oil
1/4 cup balsamic vinegar
1 tablespoon honey
Salt and pepper to taste

DIRECTIONS

- Preheat the oven to 400°F (200°C).
- Add salt, pepper, and olive oil to Brussels sprouts and toss.
- Place the Brussels sprouts on a baking sheet in just one layer.
- Roast for 15-20 minutes, or until tender and slightly browned.
- While the Brussels sprouts roast, whisk together balsamic vinegar and honey in a small saucepan.
- Bring the balsamic mixture to a simmer and cook for 5-7 minutes, or until slightly thickened.
- Drizzle the balsamic glaze over the roasted Brussels sprouts before serving.

NUTRITIONAL VALUE (APPROXIMATE):
- Calories: 150
- Protein: 2g
- Fat: 10g (healthy fats from olive oil)
- Carbs: 15g (fiber: 3g)

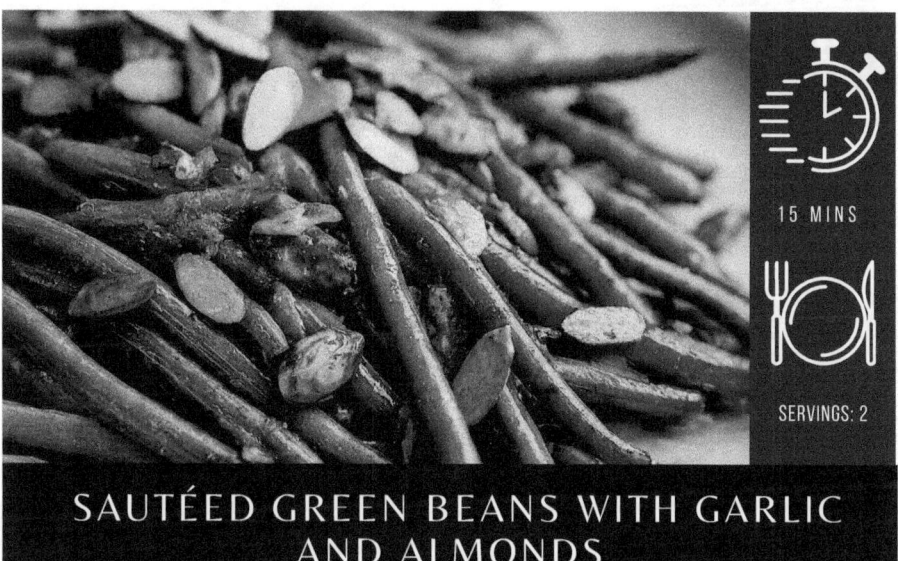

15 MINS

SERVINGS: 2

SAUTÉED GREEN BEANS WITH GARLIC AND ALMONDS

INGREDIENTS

- 1 pound fresh green beans, trimmed
- 1 tablespoon olive oil
- 2 cloves garlic, minced
- 1/4 cup sliced almonds
- Salt and pepper to taste

DIRECTIONS

1. Wash and trim the green beans. If desired, chop them into pieces that are bite-sized.
2. In a big skillet over moderate heat, warm up the olive oil.
3. Sauté the garlic for 30 seconds, or until it becomes aromatic.
4. Add green beans and cook for 5-7 minutes, or until tender-crisp.
5. Stir in sliced almonds and cook for an additional minute.
6. Season with salt and pepper to taste.

NUTRITIONAL VALUE(APPROXIMATE):

- Calories: 150
- Protein: 4g
- Fat: 10g (healthy fats from olive oil and almonds)
- Carbs: 10g (fiber: 2g)

Steamed Asparagus with Lemon and Herbs

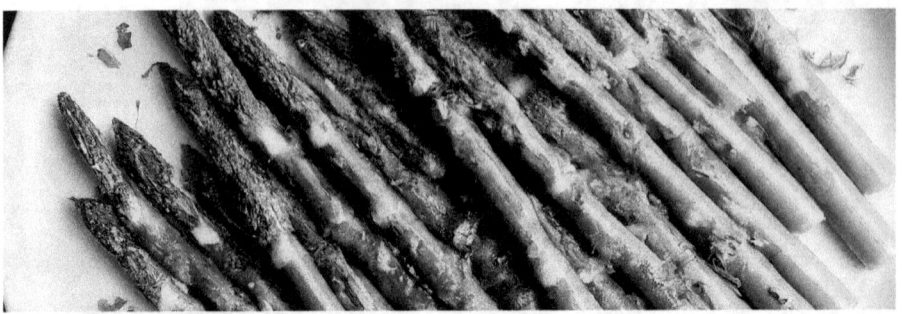

Ingredients:

- 1 pound fresh asparagus, trimmed
- 1/2 cup water
- 1 tablespoon lemon juice
- 1 teaspoon chopped fresh herbs (parsley, dill, or thyme)
- Salt and pepper to taste

Instructions:

- Wash and trim the asparagus.
- In a steamer basket, arrange the asparagus spears.
- Fill a pot with 1/2 cup of water and bring to a boil.
- Place the steamer basket over the boiling water and cover.
- Steam the asparagus for 5-7 minutes, or until tender-crisp.
- While the asparagus steams, mix lemon juice and chopped herbs in a small bowl.
- Drizzle the lemon herb mixture over the cooked asparagus and season with salt and pepper to taste.

Nutritional Value (Approximate):

- Calories: 50
- Protein: 2g
- Fat: 0g
- Carbs: 5g (fiber: 1g)

Servings: 2

Preparation time : 12 mins

Roasted Butternut Squash with Cinnamon and Pecans

 2 servings   45 minutes

INGREDIENTS

1 medium butternut squash, peeled and cubed
1 tablespoon olive oil
1/2 teaspoon ground cinnamon
1/4 cup chopped pecans
Salt and pepper to taste

DIRECTIONS

1. Preheat oven to 400°F (200°C).
2. Toss cubed butternut squash with olive oil, cinnamon, salt, and pepper.
3. Distribute the squash in a single layer on a baking pan.
4. Roast for 25-30 minutes, or until tender and slightly browned, stirring occasionally.
5. In the last 5 minutes of roasting, sprinkle the chopped pecans over the butternut squash and continue baking until the pecans are toasted.

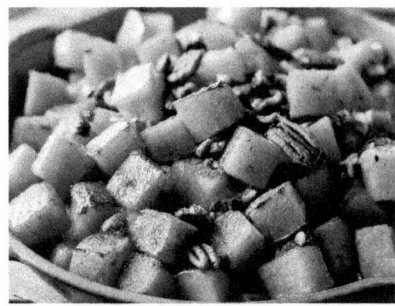

NUTRITIONAL VALUE (APPROXIMATE)
- Calories: 200
- Protein: 2g
- Fat: 12g (healthy fats from olive oil and pecans)
- Carbs: 20g (fiber: 5g)

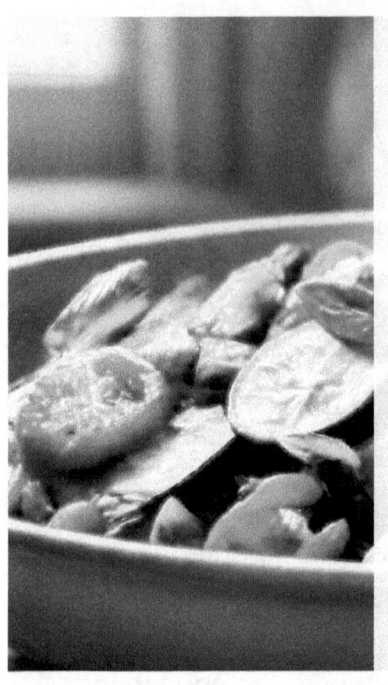

Sauteed Zucchini with Tomatoes and Basil

 2 servings   15 minutes

INGREDIENTS

1 medium zucchini, sliced
1 tablespoon olive oil
1 roma tomato, diced
2 cloves garlic, minced
1/4 cup chopped fresh basil
Salt and pepper to taste

DIRECTIONS

- Wash and slice the zucchini.
- In a big skillet over moderately high heat, warm up the olive oil.
- Fry the garlic for 30 seconds, or until it becomes flavorful.
- Add zucchini and cook for 5-7 minutes, or until tender-crisp.
- Stir in diced tomatoes and cook for an additional minute.
- Add chopped basil and cook for another minute, or until fragrant.
- Season with salt and pepper to taste.

NUTRITIONAL VALUE (APPROXIMATE):

- Calories: 100
- Protein: 1g
- Fat: 5g (healthy fats from olive oil)
- Carbs: 10g (fiber: 2g)

Chapter 7: 7-Day Sample Meal Plan

Day 1

- Breakfast: Berry Chia Seed Pudding
- Lunch: Tuna Salad with Whole-Wheat Pita and Vegetables
- Dinner: Baked Salmon with Roasted Asparagus and Quinoa
- Snack: Apple Slices with Almond Butter

Day 2

- Breakfast: High-Fiber Oatmeal with Apples and Cinnamon
- Lunch: Greek Chicken Salad with Whole-Wheat Wrap
- Dinner: Turkey Meatloaf with Mashed Cauliflower
- Snack: Cottage Cheese with Berries and Chia Seeds

Day 3

- Breakfast: Scrambled Eggs with Avocado and Tomatoes
- Lunch: Lentil Soup with Whole-Wheat Toast

- Dinner: Chicken Stir-Fry with Brown Rice and Vegetables
- Snack: Roasted Chickpeas with Spices

Day 4

- Breakfast: Whole-Wheat Toast with Smoked Salmon and Cream Cheese
- Lunch: Quinoa Salad with Roasted Vegetables
- Dinner: Vegetarian Chili with Quinoa and Black Beans
- Snack: Greek Yogurt with Sliced Banana and Walnuts

Day 5

- Breakfast: Spicy Veggie Frittata
- Lunch: Edamame Bowl with Brown Rice and Vegetables
- Dinner: Lentil and Vegetable Soup with Whole-Wheat Bread
- Snack: Edamame Pods with Sea Salt

Day 6

- Breakfast: Baked Apples with Cinnamon and Walnuts
- Lunch: Arugula Salad with Pears, Walnuts, and Blue Cheese

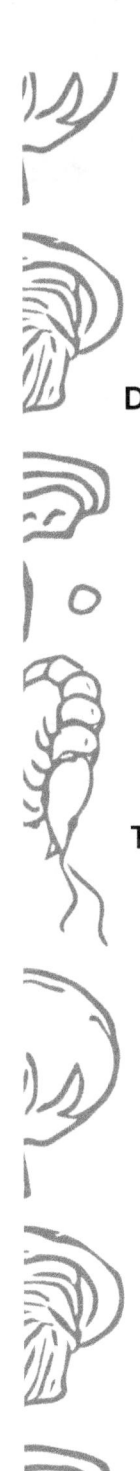

- Dinner: Baked Cod with Lemon and Herbs
- Snack: Dates with Nut Butter and Dark Chocolate

Day 7

- Breakfast: Pan-Seared Salmon with Garlic and Spinach
- Lunch: Greek Salad with Grilled Chicken and Lemon Oregano Vinaigrette
- Dinner: Mediterranean Chickpea Stew with Tomatoes and Spinach
- Snack: Frozen Banana "Nice Cream"

TIP

- Prepare some meals in advance, such as chopping vegetables or cooking quinoa, to save time during the week.

Bonus: Free Audio Version

Scan code to get access to the audio version of this book

21-Day Meal Planner

DAILY MEAL PLANNER

DAY/DATE: _____

BREAKFAST

LUNCH

DINNER

SNACKS

GROCERY LIST

NOTES

DAILY MEAL PLANNER

DAY/DATE: _____

BREAKFAST

LUNCH

DINNER

SNACKS

GROCERY LIST

NOTES

DAILY MEAL PLANNER

DAY/DATE: _____

BREAKFAST

LUNCH

DINNER

SNACKS

GROCERY LIST

NOTES

DAILY MEAL PLANNER

DAY/DATE: _____

BREAKFAST

LUNCH

DINNER

SNACKS

GROCERY LIST

NOTES

DAILY MEAL PLANNER

DAY/DATE: _____

BREAKFAST

LUNCH

DINNER

SNACKS

GROCERY LIST

NOTES

DAILY MEAL PLANNER

DAY/DATE: _____

BREAKFAST

LUNCH

DINNER

SNACKS

GROCERY LIST

NOTES
_____
_____
_____
_____

DAILY MEAL PLANNER

DAY/DATE: _____

BREAKFAST

LUNCH

DINNER

SNACKS

GROCERY LIST

NOTES

DAILY MEAL PLANNER

DAY/DATE: _____

BREAKFAST

LUNCH

DINNER

SNACKS

GROCERY LIST

NOTES

DAILY MEAL PLANNER

DAY/DATE: _____

BREAKFAST

LUNCH

DINNER

SNACKS

GROCERY LIST

NOTES

DAILY MEAL PLANNER

DAY/DATE: _____

BREAKFAST

LUNCH

DINNER

SNACKS

GROCERY LIST

NOTES
_____
_____
_____
_____

DAILY MEAL PLANNER

DAY/DATE: _____

BREAKFAST

LUNCH

DINNER

SNACKS

GROCERY LIST

NOTES

DAILY MEAL PLANNER

DAY/DATE: _____

BREAKFAST

LUNCH

DINNER

SNACKS

GROCERY LIST

NOTES

DAILY MEAL PLANNER

DAY/DATE: _____

BREAKFAST

LUNCH

DINNER

SNACKS

GROCERY LIST

NOTES

DAILY MEAL PLANNER

DAY/DATE: _____

BREAKFAST

LUNCH

DINNER

SNACKS

GROCERY LIST

NOTES

DAILY MEAL PLANNER

DAY/DATE: _____

BREAKFAST

GROCERY LIST

LUNCH

DINNER

SNACKS

NOTES

DAILY MEAL PLANNER

DAY/DATE: _____

BREAKFAST

LUNCH

DINNER

SNACKS

GROCERY LIST

NOTES

DAILY MEAL PLANNER

DAY/DATE: _____

BREAKFAST

LUNCH

DINNER

SNACKS

GROCERY LIST

NOTES

DAILY MEAL PLANNER

DAY/DATE: _____

BREAKFAST

LUNCH

DINNER

SNACKS

GROCERY LIST

NOTES

DAILY MEAL PLANNER

DAY/DATE: _____

BREAKFAST

LUNCH

DINNER

SNACKS

GROCERY LIST

NOTES

DAILY MEAL PLANNER

DAY/DATE: _____

BREAKFAST

GROCERY LIST

LUNCH

DINNER

SNACKS

NOTES

DAILY MEAL PLANNER

DAY/DATE: _____

BREAKFAST

LUNCH

DINNER

SNACKS

GROCERY LIST

NOTES

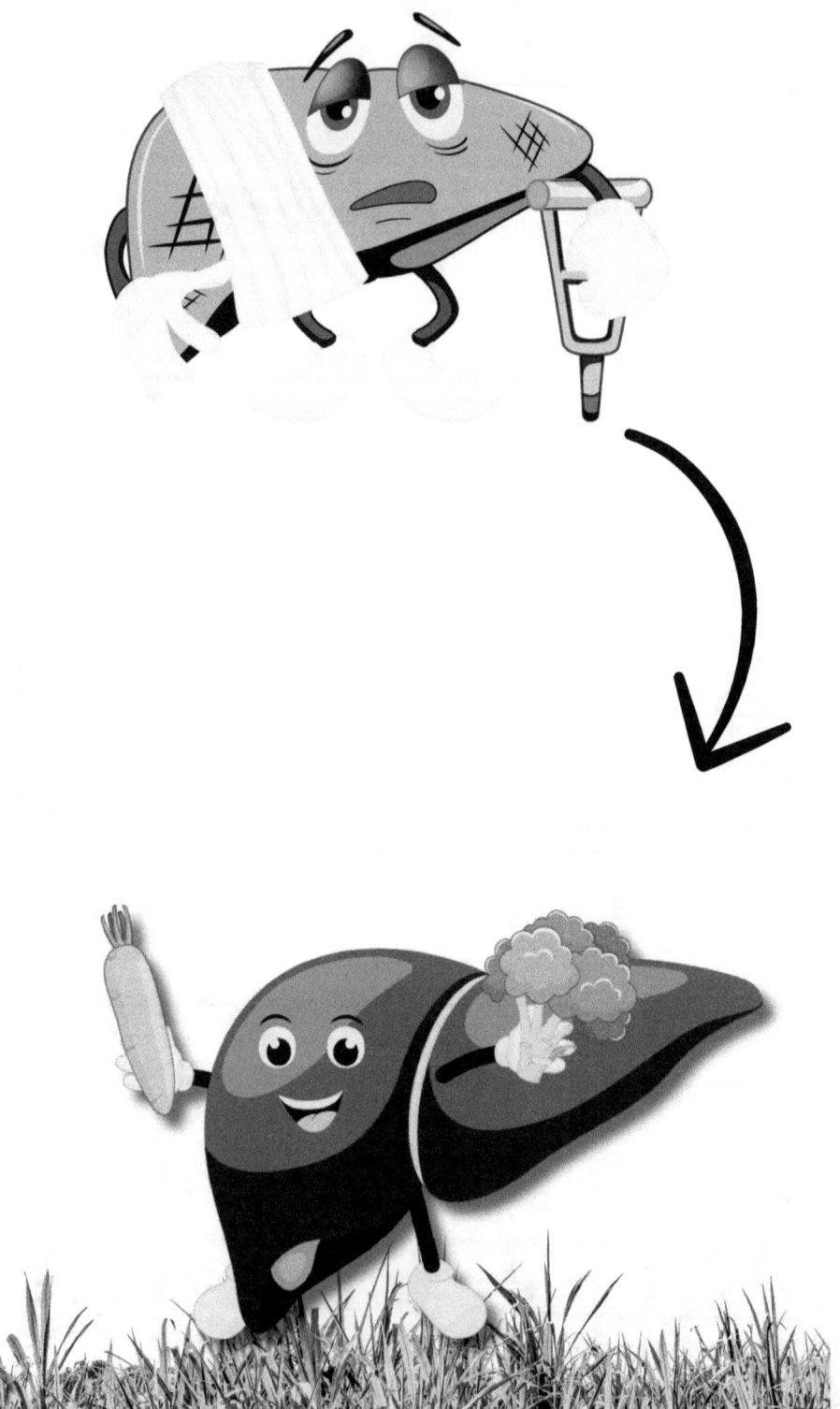

Chapter 8: Lifestyle Changes for Liver Health

Importance of Regular Exercise in Managing Liver Conditions

Your liver's a powerhouse, but even powerhouses need maintenance. That's where exercise comes in. Doc says your liver's acting up? Don't sweat it. Hit the gym, the park, anywhere you can get your blood pumping.

Exercise revs up your metabolism, burning fat that can clog your liver. Plus, it improves circulation, delivering fresh oxygen and nutrients to keep that liver functioning at peak performance. Think of it as an internal detox, naturally! So ditch the excuses and get moving. Your liver will thank you for it!

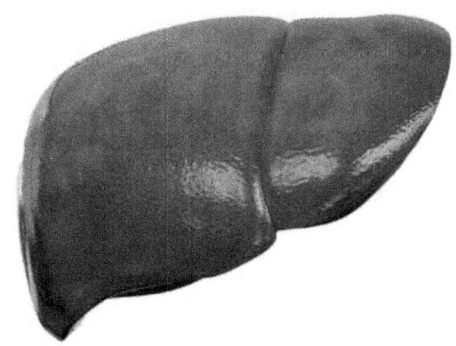

Stress Management Techniques for Liver Wellness

Chronic stress can harm your liver. Here's a stress management toolkit for your liver health:

- Mind-Body Practices: Meditation, yoga, deep breathing exercises - all help calm your nervous system and reduce stress hormones that can damage your liver.
- Adequate Sleep: Aim for 7-8 hours of quality sleep to allow your body and liver to fully repair and regenerate.
- Social Connection: Spend time with loved ones, build a support network. Strong social bonds can buffer stress and improve overall well-being.
- Organization and Planning: Feeling overwhelmed? Create schedules, to-do lists - taking control of your day can reduce stress.
- Healthy Habits: Eat a balanced diet, exercise regularly, limit alcohol - these healthy habits promote overall well-being and indirectly support liver health.

Tips for Limiting Alcohol Consumption

- Be Mindful: Pay attention to how much you're drinking and why. Are you thirsty? Celebrating? Bored? Determine the triggers and choose healthy options.
- Pace Yourself: Sip your drinks slowly and savor the flavor. Alternate alcoholic drinks with water or non-alcoholic beverages to slow down your intake.
- Plan Alcohol-Free Days: Schedule days where you abstain from alcohol completely. This gives your liver a break and helps you reset your cravings.
- Find Substitutes: Enjoy sparkling water with a lime wedge, flavorful mocktails, or
- Set SMART Goals:
    1. Specific: Aim for a specific number of drinks per day or week.
    2. Measurable: Track your drinks with a journal or app.
    3. Attainable: Start with small, achievable reductions.
    4. Relevant: Set goals that align with your overall health goals.
    5. Time-bound: Give yourself a timeframe to reach your goals.

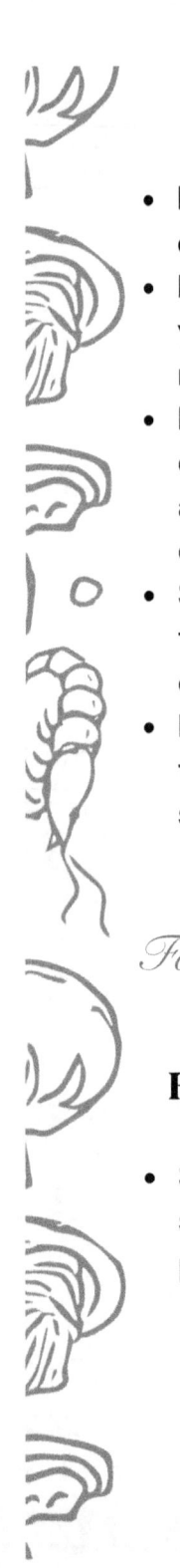

- herbal teas for a satisfying non-alcoholic drink experience.
- Listen to Your Body: Pay attention to how you feel after drinking. If you experience negative effects, it's a sign to cut back.
- Be Social Without Alcohol: Social events don't have to revolve around alcohol. Plan activities like going for a hike, playing games, or enjoying a coffee date.
- Seek Support: Talk to your doctor or a trusted friend about your goals. They can offer encouragement and resources.
- Reward Yourself: Celebrate your progress towards your goals! Treat yourself to something non-alcoholic you enjoy.

Foods and fruits to take and to avoid

Foods to Avoid:

- Sugary Drinks and Foods: These include soda, juice, sweetened coffee drinks, pastries, candy, and sugary cereals. They

contribute to high blood sugar and excess fat storage in the liver.
- Red Meat and Processed Meats: High in saturated fat, which can worsen fatty liver disease. Limit red meat and avoid processed meats like bacon, sausage, and hot dogs. Also avoid the skin of poultry.
- Fried Foods: High in unhealthy fats and calories, increasing stress on the liver. Select healthier cooking techniques such as steaming, grilling, or oven baking.
- Refined Grains: White bread, pasta, and rice can cause blood sugar spikes. Choose whole grains instead, like brown rice, quinoa, and whole-wheat bread.
- Salty Foods: Excessive sodium can lead to fluid retention and potentially worsen liver complications. Limit processed foods, canned goods, and added table salt.

Fruits to Limit:

- Fructose-Rich Fruits: While fruit is generally healthy, some are higher in fructose, a sugar processed by the liver. Limit fruits like grapes, mangoes, and pears.
- Dried Fruits: Often concentrated in sugar content compared to fresh fruit. Opt for fresh fruits or limit dried fruit portions.

Foods and fruits to take:

Fruits

- Low-Fructose Fruits: Choose fruits lower in fructose, which the liver processes. Great options include berries (blueberries, raspberries, strawberries), cranberries, apples, grapefruits, and kiwis.
- Whole Fruits Over Juices: Opt for whole fruits over juices to benefit from fiber, vitamins, and minerals, and avoid concentrated sugar intake.

Vegetables

- Leafy Greens: Powerhouses of vitamins, minerals, and antioxidants. Include spinach, kale, Swiss chard, romaine lettuce, and collard greens.
- Cruciferous Vegetables: Broccoli, cauliflower, Brussels sprouts, and cabbage are rich in antioxidants and phytonutrients that support liver health.
- Other Colorful Vegetables: Explore a variety of colors for a diverse nutrient intake. Include carrots, sweet potatoes, beets, bell peppers, and asparagus.

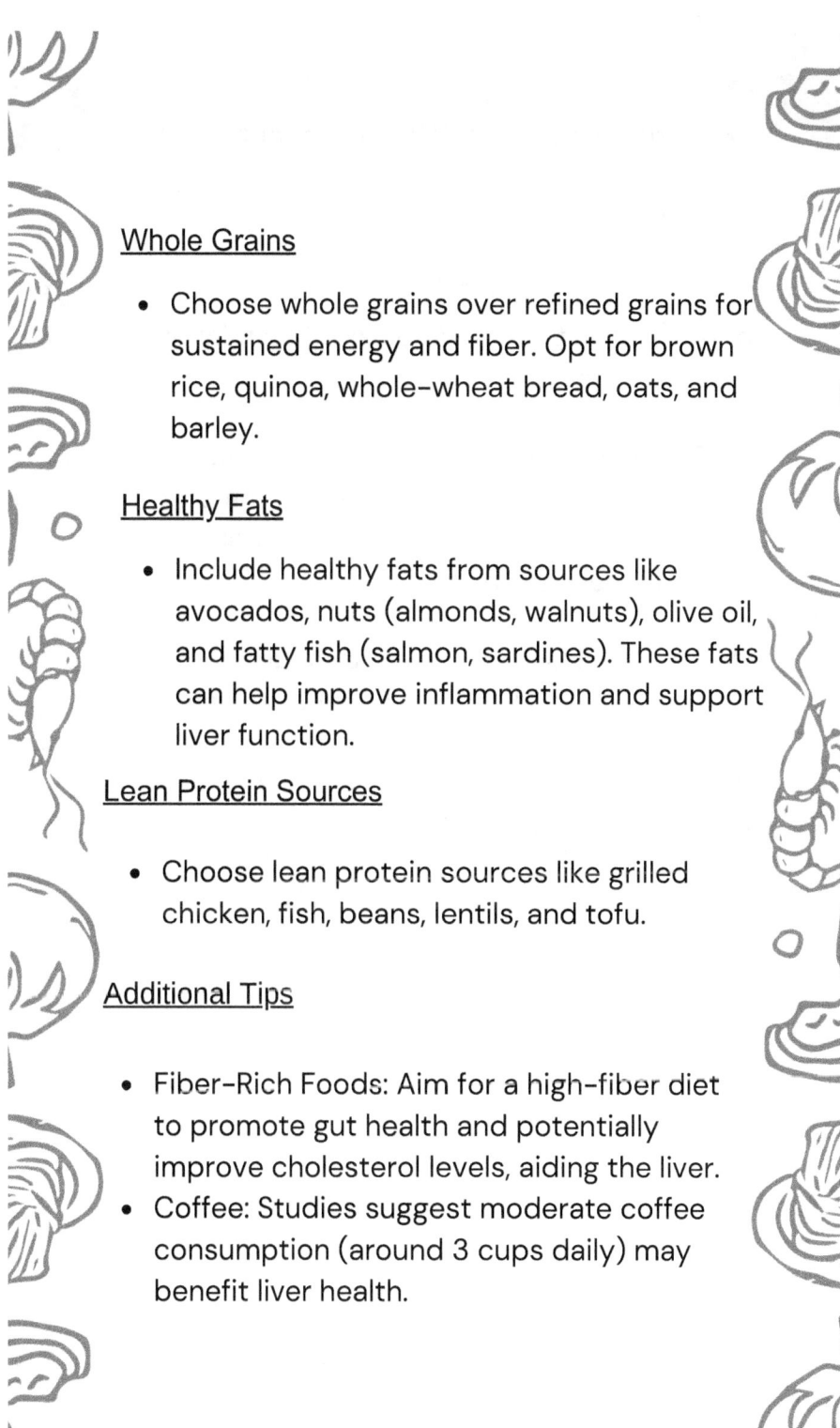

Whole Grains

- Choose whole grains over refined grains for sustained energy and fiber. Opt for brown rice, quinoa, whole-wheat bread, oats, and barley.

Healthy Fats

- Include healthy fats from sources like avocados, nuts (almonds, walnuts), olive oil, and fatty fish (salmon, sardines). These fats can help improve inflammation and support liver function.

Lean Protein Sources

- Choose lean protein sources like grilled chicken, fish, beans, lentils, and tofu.

Additional Tips

- Fiber-Rich Foods: Aim for a high-fiber diet to promote gut health and potentially improve cholesterol levels, aiding the liver.
- Coffee: Studies suggest moderate coffee consumption (around 3 cups daily) may benefit liver health.

- Dandelion root tea: Dandelion root is a natural diuretic that may help stimulate bile production and elimination of toxins.

How to Use: Steep 1-2 teaspoons of dried dandelion root in hot water for 10-15 minutes. Strain and enjoy.

- Turmeric golden milk: Turmeric contains curcumin, a powerful anti-inflammatory compound with liver-protective benefits. Black pepper enhances curcumin absorption.

How to Use: Combine 1 teaspoon turmeric powder, 1 cup milk (dairy or non-dairy), and a pinch of black pepper in a saucepan. Heat gently, whisking frequently, until warmed through. Do not boil. Enjoy warm.

- Water: Stay hydrated with plenty of water throughout the day to support overall health and liver function.
- Low sodium foods: Intake of foods low in sodium can help reduce fluid build up in the liver . However when the level of sodium in your body system is too low it can cause muscle cramps, nausea and dizziness so don't take it in excess

<u>Remember</u>

- Adjust portion sizes based on your calorie requirements.

Natural Methods to Detoxify the Liver

- Milk thistle extract/supplements: Milk thistle has been used for centuries to support liver health. It contains silymarin, a group of antioxidants that may help protect liver cells from damage.

How to Use: Similar to dandelion root tea, you can brew a tea using 1-2 teaspoons of crushed milk thistle seeds steeped in hot water for 10-15 minutes. Strain and enjoy.

- Dandelion root tea: Dandelion root is a natural diuretic that may help stimulate bile production and elimination of toxins.

How to Use: Steep 1-2 teaspoons of dried dandelion root in hot water for 10-15 minutes. Strain and enjoy.

- Turmeric golden milk: Turmeric contains curcumin, a powerful anti-inflammatory compound with liver-protective benefits. Black pepper enhances curcumin absorption.

How to Use: Combine 1 teaspoon turmeric powder, 1 cup milk (dairy or non-dairy), and a pinch of black pepper in a saucepan. Heat gently, whisking frequently, until warmed through. Do not boil. Enjoy warm.

- Proper hydration: Drinking plenty of water helps flush toxins from your body and keeps your liver functioning optimally.

How to Use: Aim to drink throughout the day. There are different recommendations on the amount of water needed, but a good rule of thumb is to drink when you feel thirsty.

- Olive oil: Olive oil is a healthy fat that may improve liver function and reduce inflammation.

How to Use: Use olive oil for cooking or drizzling on salads.

- Green tea: Green tea is rich in antioxidants that may protect the liver from damage.

How to Use: Steep 1 green tea bag in hot water for 3-5 minutes. Strain and enjoy.

- Garlic infusion: Garlic has detoxifying properties and may help support liver health.

How to Use: Crush 1-2 garlic cloves and steep them in hot water for 10 minutes. Strain and enjoy.

- Fresh beetroot juice: Beetroot juice is a good source of antioxidants and nitrates, which may help improve blood flow and detoxification in the liver.

How to Use: Extract juice from fresh beetroot and consume. You can also add beetroot to smoothies or soups.

Conversion chart

Equivalency Chart

Cup	Fluid Oz	Tablespoon	Teaspoon	Milliliter
1 cup	8 oz	16 tbsp	48 tsp	237 ml
3/4 cup	6 oz	12 tbsp	36 tsp	177 ml
2/3 cup	5 oz	9 tbsp	27 tsp	158 ml
1/2 cup	4 oz	8 tbsp	24 tsp	118 ml
1/3 cup	3 oz	5 tbsp	16 tsp	79 ml
1/4 cup	2 oz	4 tbsp	12 tsp	59 ml
1/8 cup	1 oz	2 tbsp	6 tsp	30 ml
1/16 cup	1/2 oz	1 tbsp	3 tsp	15 ml

Cups	Fluid Oz	Pint	Quart	Gallon
16 cups	128 oz	8 pt	4 qt	1 gal
8 cups	64 oz	4 pt	2 qt	1/2 gal
4 cups	32 oz	2 pt	1 qt	1/4 gal
2 cups	16 oz	1 pt	1/2 qt	1/8 gal
1 cup	8 oz	1/2 pt	1/4 qt	1/16 gal

Conclusion

We've covered a lot of ground in this book. You've learned the lingo, faced the fatty liver facts, and most importantly, discovered a toolbox full of delicious recipes to keep your liver happy.
Focus on real, unprocessed foods. Fill your plate with colorful veggies, lean protein, and healthy fats. Don't forget the fiber from whole grains to keep your system movin' and groovin'.
And remember, sugar and processed junk? Those are the enemies. Keep 'em at bay, and your liver will thank you for it.

Exercise is your partner in crime. Get your heart rate up, break a sweat. It helps your body process nutrients better, taking the pressure off your liver. Finally, ditch the booze or cut back drastically. Alcohol is the public enemy number one.
This ain't a one-time fix. It's a lifestyle shift, a commitment to your health. But trust me, with these tips and these tasty recipes, you'll be feeling good and supporting your liver function in no time. You got this!

Remember, knowledge is power, and you've got the knowledge to rock a healthy liver and a life that feels freakin' fantastic! Now get out there, make those recipes, and show your liver some love.

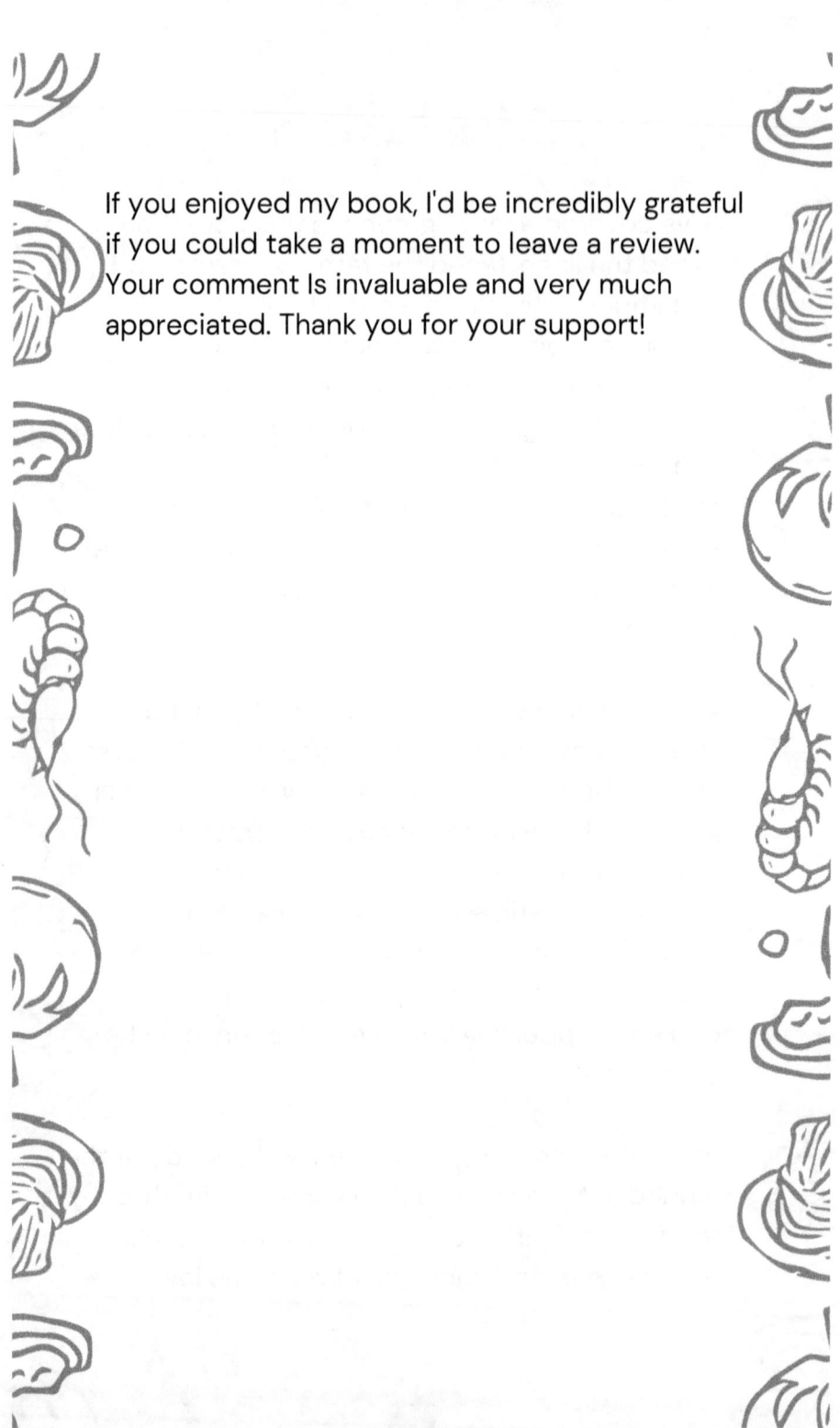

If you enjoyed my book, I'd be incredibly grateful if you could take a moment to leave a review. Your comment Is invaluable and very much appreciated. Thank you for your support!

www.ingramcontent.com/pod-product-compliance
Lightning Source LLC
Chambersburg PA
CBHW050311230526
45471CB00005B/2122